Health, Art & Reason

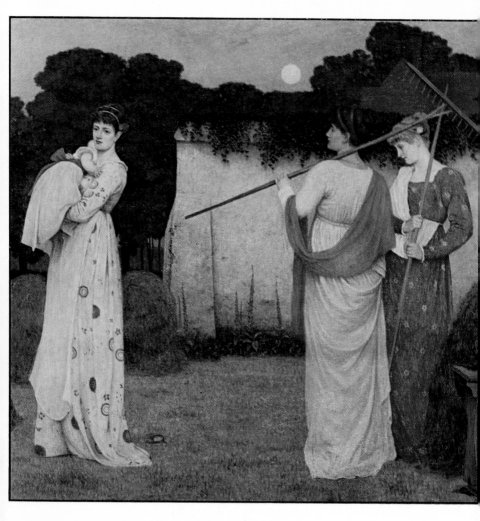

'Haytime (The Hayfield).' Thomas Armstrong

Health, Art & Reason

DRESS REFORMERS OF THE 19TH CENTURY

Stella Mary Newton

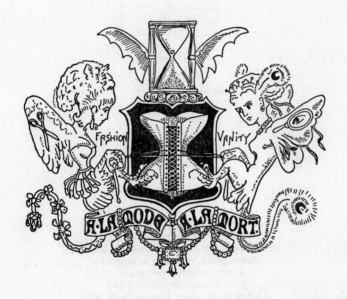

JOHN MURRAY

Printed in Great Britain by
Cox & Wyman Ltd
London, Fakenham and Reading

0 7195 2424 5

To ANGUS ACWORTH CBE
in gratitude for the help and encouragement
he has given me in my study
of the history of dress

Contents

Illustrations

Illustrations

(See Appendix 2 for details of line illustrations at the beginning of each chapter)

Acknowledgement is due to the following for permission to reproduce illustrations in this book or for supplying photographs.

Victoria and Albert Museum, frontispiece and jacket, 1, 3; British Museum, 2; Makins Collection, 6; Fitzwilliam Museum, Cambridge, 7; Gernsheim Collection, University of Texas, 8; National Trust, 9; Louvre, 14, 15; Mansell/Alinari, 18; Burlington Magazine, 26; Art Institute of Chicago, 30; Jaeger Ltd, 37, 38; Glen Byam Shaw, 56; Watts Gallery and Ronald Chapman, 58; Olivier Rouart, 61; Elsevier Publishers, Brussels, 62.

Numbers in square brackets refer to the illustrations to be found between pp. 20–21 and pp. 100–101

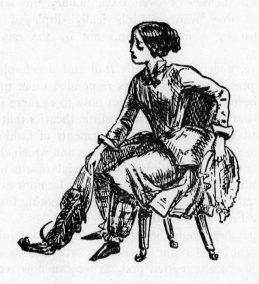

1

Women with Views

Artistic, hygienic, rational are not among today's most familiar adjectives; philosophers, novelists and advertising copy-writers can get along very well without them. The phenomena they helped to describe belonged to the 19th century not to ours. The urge to distinguish the well-designed exceptions from the mass of ugly trivia displayed in the Great Exhibition of 1851 had produced the adjective 'artistic'; 'hygienic' arrived as a result of the missionary fight against the overcrowding and the cholera invasions of the middle decades of the 19th century; 'rational' achieved popularity in the effort to substitute clear and simple thinking for muddled verbosity.

I

This book is a study of fashionable dress – a parable in which the concepts 'artistic', 'hygienic', 'rational' found circulation. Since the ideas themselves were revolutionary the fashions through which they were metaphorically displayed were, naturally, worn by a minority and not by the establishment.

By its nature, which is essentially frail and perishable, the dress of the upper-classes has always responded more quickly than any of the other applied arts not only to changes in the social pattern but even to the first idealistic theories that have preceded them. Within the larger movements of fashion, to which in the long run all artifacts are subject and which change at a pace fitting to the more permanent materials of which most works of art and craftsmanship are composed, fashions in dress revolve like small eddies in a larger current, exposing first one aspect of prevailing taste and then another.

Nothing, therefore, could better exemplify the intensity of the mid-19th century's fervour for social reform than its attack on the concept of fashion itself and, as we can now see, the inevitable result was the creation of new fashions. But the attack was courageous and, if not unique in history, was among the very few recorded instances of an attempt to demolish this basic principle of civilisation.

Even in their earliest attempts to replace what they regarded as unhealthy, inartistic and ridiculous fashions in dress, reformers were aware that fashion extended into other forms of human expression as well, but the evils of fashionable clothing, especially that of females, seemed the most urgently in need of reform on hygienic, artistic and rational lines.

In 1850 the unease which was to call these three words into use was already stirring in the ground; by 1870 the new ideas had pushed their way up and through the surface to be recognised as important by the kind of people who look out intelligently for new things; in full flower in the 1880s – that most earnest of decades – everybody who read the papers knew about them though most people did not care for their aroma. Despised as already *vieux jeu* by the restless fashionable world of the 'nineties they were, at the same time, recommended as desirable for the working-classes. The First World War of the 20th century killed and buried them.

The exact form of their germination in the 1850s was unexpected and, to those who had been fostering them, must have been disturbing for, very early in that decade young and pretty Mrs Dexter C. Bloomer of New York devised and adopted for her own dress, a type of suit that was soon named after her – the Bloomer. This dress which was also adopted by some American women who shared Amelia Bloomer's views on the emancipation of women, consisted of ankle-length, baggy trousers, worn beneath a loose tunic which reached to, or a little below, the knee.[1]

Mrs Bloomer certainly had both hygiene and common sense in mind when she sought to establish her suit as a substitute for the normal feminine dress of the end of the 1840s which involved several layers of heavy under-petticoats to give it the bulk required by fashion. As for its being artistic, although she did not, in all probability, apply the term to her new dress even to herself, she undoubtedly intended it to be attractive.

Mrs Bloomer was, throughout her life, an active champion of the emancipation of women. In later life she denied that her Bloomer had ever played an important part in her campaigns for their Rights and she gave it up, she said, when, in the later 1850s, comfortable crinolines replaced heavy petticoats and when, moving with her husband to a windy part of the United States, the short skirt she wore with her Bloomer blew up embarrassingly over her head.[2]

In the early years of the 1850s, before the invention of the crinoline under-cage, Mrs Bloomer defended with wit the costume she had invented. When a Reverend Mr Talmadge quoted Moses from the pulpit as the authority who had forbidden women to wear men's clothes, her comment was that the first fashion was set by Adam and Eve when they assumed fig-leaves, and nowhere was it stated that while Adam's were bifurcated Eve's were not. The second fashion, she went on, was set by God himself when he clothed them both in skins;

but there was no indication that there had been any difference in design between the two.[3]

Mrs Bloomer would probably never have arrived at her design for the Bloomer at all if it had not been for the numerous popular engravings of melting beauties in Turkish trousers that followed the cult of Byron and the French conquest of Algeria. [2] As heroines of poems, songs and short stories in women's magazines, these western nieces of Delacroix's *Algeriennes* with their huge eyes and tiny waists lounged seductively but with decency in unconventional poses on the ground, showing delicious little feet. Seduction was not absent from the Bloomer costume; in describing its pantaloons Mrs Bloomer insisted that they should reach the ankle but not the instep and that when they were worn with boots these should be, 'gracefully sloped on the upper edge and trimmed with fur or fancifully embroidered'.[4] The pantaloons were to be looseish and held in at the ankle by elastic; the coat worn over them was to have a full skirt and reach to about, or a little below, the knee. It was this skirt which, Mrs Bloomer discovered, blew up so inconveniently on a windy day. From one engraving that survives it is difficult to see Mrs Bloomer as in any way mannish. [1]

English women of the 1850s were certainly amused as well as shocked by the Bloomer but they did not for a moment think of wearing it. Between 1851 and 1853 it was thoroughly explored as a theme for jokes in *Punch*, [4] but apart from these its most immediate result in England seems to have been to give birth to a music-hall song. This must have had some popularity for *I'll be a Bloomer* appeared first with the engraving – hand-coloured – of Mrs Bloomer on its cover and was later issued as a single song-sheet headed by a stock design of a run-of-the-mill ballet dancer with little wings:

> Listen females all,
> No matter what your trade is,
> Old Nick is in the girls
> The d——l's in the ladies;

Married men may weep
    And tumble in the ditches
Since women are resolved,
    To wear the shirt and breeches.

Ladies do declare,
    A change should have been sooner
The women one and all
    Are going to join the Bloomers,

Prince Albert and the Queen,
    Had such a jolly row, sirs,
She threw off the stays and put
    On waistcoat, coat and trousers.

These are the first of the twenty-two verses which end with:

Yankee Doodle doo,
    Rolling in the ditches
Married men prepare
    To buy your women the breeches.[5]

In due course the Bloomer, which enjoyed a small *succès de scandale* in the United States, had attracted so much public attention in England that in 1857 the novelist Charles Reade centred the plot of a novelette, *The Course of True Love never did Run Smooth*, round his heroine, Caroline Courtney, a young American who wore the Bloomer. By this time it had been, or was about to be, abandoned as a costume by Mrs Bloomer herself.

Charles Reade presented his Caroline Courtney as a serious-minded young woman who saw herself not only as an emulator but as a disciple of Mrs Bloomer:

A polka concluded, a tide of servants poured in. A semi-circle of seats sprung up – A pulpit rose like an exhalation and almost before her guests could seat themselves, Caroline was a lecturer wearing over her Bloomer a B.C.L. gown from

Oxford and the four-cornered cap of that University on her head.[6]

The cover of Charles Reade's *The Course of True Love never did Run Smooth* shows the heroine, Caroline, in neat tapering trousers and a knee-length coat looking rather like the young Chopin and considerably more boyish than Amelia Bloomer. [3] Apart from her championship of the Bloomer, Caroline is interesting as probably the first of the long line of young and beautiful American heiresses of 19th-century fiction – desirable, innocent, high-spirited girls of whose families, by good or ill fortune, no member ever survived to play the restraining role of chaperone. And like most of them Caroline had a handsome young English aristocrat at her feet – Reginald Seymour.

Reade's Caroline Courtney nearly lost her Reginald in her headstrong determination to wear the Bloomer. As she descended the pulpit after delivering her sermon in its defence she caught a glimpse through a window of his ship sailing for home and fainted at the sight. When, soon afterwards, she followed him to England, she was presented, wearing her Bloomer, with the opportunity of rescuing him from drowning in an English stream, an undertaking that would have been impossible, apparently, in the fashionable crinoline. Although in his gratitude Reginald Seymour was almost reconciled to the hated Bloomer, Caroline revealed that she had only put it on for one last time to tease him.[7]

In introducing the rescue incident Charles Reade was daring. It was not easy to defend the Bloomer in America in 1857, much less in England; what were probably Reade's real views on the subject were spoken not by his hero and heroine but by one of his low-class minor characters. The servants who had 'poured in' to hear Caroline's lecture had already discussed the Bloomer below stairs in the kitchen. The story, written partly in dramatic dialogue in a style for which unconventional is too mild a word, is at its most farouche in the scene between Elisa, the cook, and Caroline's maid Angelina, admired by Giles, 'a Briton in the suite of young Seymour', with Mrs Trimmer, the housekeeper as arbitrator. Elisa, who is making pastry, declares that she means to wear the Bloomer, but only she of the four can bring herself to mention it by name.

Angelina: Well I think a Woman should dress to gratify the men (with an oeillard at Giles) not to imitate them.

Elisa: The men! so long as we sweep the streets for them with our skirts, they are all right. You talk of delicacy, is dirt delicacy?

On this she whipped off a chair by the fire a gown that had met with a misfortune: it had been out walking on a wet day. Elisa put it viciously under Angelina's nose who recoiled. An accurate description of it would soil these pages.

'Is that pretty,' continued the cook, 'to carry a hundred weight of muck wherever you go?'

'Dirt can't be helped,' retorted Trimmer. 'Indecency can.'

'Indecent!' cried Elisa with a face like scarlet, 'who's a going to be indecent in this kitchen?'

'The gals,' suggested Angelina, 'who wear – who wear—'

'Small clothes,' put in Giles.

A grateful glance repaid him for extricating the pair from a conventional difficulty.

'What, its indecent because it shows your instep I suppose? You go into the drawing-room this evening and the young ladies shall show you more than ever a Bloomer will. Women's delicacy!' said Elisa, putting her hand under the paste on the table and bringing it down with a whack 'Gammon! Fashion is what we care for, not delicacy. If it was the fashion to tie our right foot to our left ear wouldn't you do it?'

'No!' said Angelina with but little hesitation.[8]

In this scene, which posed the problem of both the irrationality of fashion and the insanitary nature of women's clothes, the author appeared as a prophet; ten years later, at the end of the 1860s, the sentiments which he had put into the mouths of his low-comedy servants were to occupy loftier minds with increasing frequency. He had been alone in seeing the dress devised by Amelia Bloomer as an advance in the direction of hygiene, and his recognition of the connection between female emancipation and the health of the community must have passed unnoticed for *the Course of True Love* was soon forgotten – the theme of the little story had been topical, its philosophy was uttered too soon.

Light-hearted and silly as it was, *The Course of True Love* included another topic of growing concern at the time of its publication, which Reade also contrived to illustrate by references to dress – the intellectual capabilities of women. When she mounted her pulpit wearing a graduate's gown (borrowed from Reginald) over her Bloomer, Caroline Courtney made it clear that she was not uneducated. Accompanied by cords struck on a piano to serve as punctuation, she introduced in recitative and verse the members of her cast, all of whom wore styles of dress both ugly and ephemeral, representing fashions of the past, then in contrast, she invoked peasants from Armenia, Poland and Sicily in their unchanging regional types of dress. Her aim was to emphasise the point that, whether ugly or beautiful:

> Such fashions are like poppies spread
> You seize the flower, the bloom is fled:
> Or like a snowflake on a river
> A moment seen, then gone forever.[9]

Caroline Courtney's entertainment continued with the appearance of two Persian ladies in 'pantaloons', declaiming:

> Three revolutions of the moon are completed since we sailed in ships from Istamboul; in the meantime Sheitan has doubtless obtained permission to derange this people's intellects, so that they may be converted to the true faith . . .

They called upon the 'Holy Prophet' to witness the madness of the customs of western women (providing, incidentally, a link between the Bloomer and Turkish dress). Finally Caroline ordered her cook – who was incapable of doing so – to pronounce the words; 'Adsis, O Cato'; whereupon Cato, 'swept in' in a skirt-like toga, Crying; 'Adsum, quis me vocat?'[10]

Ephemeral but significant, Amelia Bloomer's romantic design for an emancipated dress attempted, though she may not have thought in precisely those terms, to show that beauty and utility were not incompatible and that women should be allowed not only the first but the second too. Charles Reade saw what she had done and added a further emphasis in pointing out that no absolute existed in the design of dress for whereas Turkish women, whose main – virtually *only* – function was feminity, wore trousers, Roman patricians, even the most noble and courageous of them, wore skirts.

Caroline's whole performance was conceived by the author at the moment when crinolines were at their widest – the end of the 'fifties, so that in ridiculing the whole concept of fashion this aspect of it naturally influenced his choice. When, for instance, Caroline added a further dramatic scene to her party by conjuring-up a procession of women wearing dresses of the historic past, Queen Elizabeth I appeared the most disastrous in her dress. He declared:

Set a stomacher three feet long between two monstrous jelly-bags upon a bloated bell and there you have this queen and her successor in New York

While Caroline's comment was:

common-sense fell flatter than Spain the day that Royalty appeared thus

She refrained from adding that the reigning queen of England did not dress so very differently. She demonstrated, however, that the fashions of the recent past were no less absurd, for when, wearing the straight dresses of the 'Empire' period, 'two short-waisted ladies came in' everybody burst out laughing.[11]

The dress invented by Mrs Bloomer and adopted by Caroline Courtney was never intended to look masculine. Mrs Bloomer's dress with its prototype of the trousers of Turkish ladies was definitely romantic. When he designed the cover for *the Course of True Love*, however, the English artist in presenting Caroline as a handsome youth was probably already making his own moral comment and, indeed, it was the potential masculinity of the dress which was emphasised in drawings in *Punch* and English satirical verses of the moment. Bifurcated nether garments had for so long been worn exclusively by men that Mrs Bloomer's almost light-hearted gesture in adopting them damaged the cause of female emancipation for the rest of the century.

Charles Reade was ahead of his time.[12] The theory that perfect fitness for purpose and absolute beauty of design should replace restless changes of fashion was to be propounded repeatedly by more distinguished people than Charles Reade's Caroline during the thirty years that followed her party. As what was later to be called a 'platform woman' she was not very effective but as the little heroine of an early story by a novelist who was to become eminent she was remarkable for her period. Neither Richardson's Clarissa Harlowe nor Fielding's Sophia Weston could have mounted a pulpit or issued an order in Latin before a mixed company. Now, a hundred years after their time, at the end of the 1850s, thoughtful men and women were becoming aware of the change that had taken place in the position of women even since the beginning of the 19th century – the change, too, in the attitude towards them. Women, in consequence, were beginning to see themselves in a new light.

In 1862 the *Edinburgh Review* published a long notice of a book of letters from Mrs Richard Trench, recently collected and edited by her son, the then Dean of Westminster. The reviewer's critical attitude to them is significant:

> In these our days a lady of Mrs Trench's intelligence, information and interest in all about her would have her theological and ethical speculations, her schemes of philanthropy, and her, perhaps, partial or extravagant ideas as to her duties and mission in the world. But Mrs Trench had no 'views'; she accepted without remonstrance the conditions of thought and society in which she found herself placed.[13]

Mrs Trench may have had no 'views'. She had not, presumably, been that kind of woman. But women with views had certainly existed for a long time – Judith and Delilah, not to speak of Cleopatra, certainly had some. What was new was not the existence of women with views but their ability and their liberty to express them among their friends of both sexes. For apart from the very few brilliant women of the 18th century who had established for themselves the right to invite intelligent men to meet in their drawing-rooms, most clever women of that time had spent almost all their days with members of their own sex. At the beginning of the 1860s it was this state of things that some of the clever women were trying to change and they were, for the first time, not without their male supporters.

Naturally they met with opposition. From, for instance, those men less gifted than themselves whose conversation across the billiard table or over the port, far from being highly spiced, was they must have realised, as dull and trivial as that of their wives and sisters in the drawing-room below; and from the majority of women who, like the majority of mankind at any period, either did not want to use their brains or were incapable of doing so. With the threatened advent of the 'platform woman' to join the platform man, both sexes evidently came to the conclusion that they were in danger of exposure to twice as many exhortations urging them to nurture 'theological and ethical speculations' to form 'schemes of philanthropy' and to hold 'ideas' as to their mission in the world. Of such exhortations there were, surely, enough already?

In spite, however, of opposition, a small and vocal group of determined men and women in what have been called the Serious 'Sixties were finding the means of expressing the view that women should be allowed to do some of the things hitherto reserved to men; they were not without hope of being listened to. At the beginning of the 'sixties their voices were barely raised above a whisper and the modest terms in which the women thought of themselves can be judged from, for instance, the *Owlet Papers* (fragile little feminine counterpart of the jaunty

masculine *Owl*), which addressed its readers in 1861 in the
following open letter:

> Dear Owlet, . . . Believe me, among the female section of
> society in our sphere of Graces of our time being, there is a
> brilliant but flimsy veil thrown over the statue of Ignorance.
> Every woman ought to be thoroughly informed in Grammar,
> Arithmetic, History and modern languages . . . There is
> another subject on which we would offer a word of advice,
> and that is dress. Surely it is unworthy of an intellectual
> being to be attired in a manner which precludes the possi-
> bility of almost every rational enjoyment: how is it possible
> to walk in comfort if the dress is either so long as to sweep the
> street, or, as the case is at present, so wide as to take up
> immeasurable space?[14]

But 'dear Owlet' was not advised to wear the Bloomer as
Reade's Caroline Courtney had done only three years earlier.

The tone was very different in 1868. A year previously
John Stuart Mill had proposed the equal enfranchisement of
women and men as an amendment to the Reform Bill; in
1868 *Woman's World*,[15] a weekly magazine of extremely sober
form, appeared. It included in its earlier numbers a regular
feature under the heading, The Age we Live In, which
discussed, in conversational terms, controversial questions
concerning women and challenged, in particular, many of the
opinions expressed in articles on similar aspects of the subject
which were appearing in current issues of other periodicals,
especially the *Pall Mall Gazette*.

Although *Woman's World* does not often contain specific
mention of dress, articles in its first issues throw considerable
light on the attitudes which led to dress reforms in the years to
come.

Those who spoke for The Age we Live In in *Woman's
World* were an Aunt, several of her nieces – apparently young;
the husband of one of them – John; and various subsidiary
characters who appeared now and then. All of them, except a
'Dr Caustic' who occasionally intervened, were enthusiastic

supporters of women's rights. It is typical of the period that – vociferously sympathetic to the cause though they were – it was the middle-aged Aunt, not the younger generation, who discussed the subject most lucidly, and whose penetrating judgement was always effective. It was still too early in time for the young to speak with assurance in a serious periodical.

Woman's World included, as was usual at the period, serialised novels, articles on topical sociological questions – including a regular feature called Workhouse Notes – a series of articles on Ruskin's *Stones of Venice*, and new poems. Its outlook was democratic, it eagerly supported the proposal to establish a

> Women's Social Institute for women of all ranks where they shall be free from all interference in respect to their religious opinions, but where, at the same time, the management shall be such as to secure the members from evil influence ... The working women of England are very numerous, Art students, teachers, literary women, needlewomen ...[16]

Among the latter, it was generally agreed, were the most oppressed and underpaid members of society. The institute did eventually get going in Newman Street, off Oxford Street. Like other organisations set up by women it was attacked from time to time in contemporary journals.

The article proposing the establishment of a Women's Social Institute appeared two months after *Woman's World* had published a new poem by Gerald Massey in which each verse had ended with a refrain significantly placing 'Beauty' and 'Labour' side by side:

> Then let us worship Beauty with the knightly faith of old
> O Chivalry of Labour toiling for the Age of Gold.[17]

It was an isolated plea, for *Woman's World* was not, in fact, greatly concerned with Beauty; its aim was rather to stress the importance of intellect and virtually no reference to contemporary art, even, appeared in its pages. Its chief response to

Gerald Massey's exhortation seems to have been contained in an article pressing for the admission of women to the medical profession:

> ... worship the beautiful if still you will but make way for those pale, earnest women, who desire work for some good reason, not less worthy than your own, and if she seeks it as a healer — as physician — let her pass on, offer her no hindrance ...[18]

The battle of the sexes was certainly on. In the same year the *Pall Mall Gazette* had printed a summary of an article on the Strong-minded Woman in *The Times*, saying:

> When a woman is so strong-minded as to suggest a resemblance to the stronger sex, men feel that they could not *love her,* and *accordingly do not like her*. This is a matter of instinct ...[19]

a view which *Woman's World* naturally seized on. It replied with an article called Our Place, by a Strong-minded Woman, and declared:

> I read this definition and decree of the Thunderer – once, twice, three times. ... Did the epithet Strong-minded imply strength of muscle also? Is mind muscle and muscle mind?[20]

The author went on to point out that many a man of indecisive character had been thankful to rely on the support and guidance of a wise and kindly wife – which the *Pall Mall Gazette* would probably not have denied; all it asked was that she should remain in the background, whereas *Woman's World* was determined that she should not. Whenever it had a chance, The Age we Live In discussed those women who managed to appear in public:

> 'But John, what about Miss Becker?'
> 'She has been reading a paper to the British Association, that

has quite upset the masculine equilibrium, excited the comments of all the papers, and put the *Pall Mall Gazette* in a pet.'[21]

Lydia Becker was among the small group of women who were already campaigning for the enfranchisement of their sex in the late 'sixties; she was still active twenty years later and had never ceased, in the intervening years, to fight for the cause.

Beneath all the literary sparring it is possible to see that since the beginning of the 'sixties considerable advances had been made where the position of women was concerned. Few people contributing to the thoughtful journals any longer believed that women were actually inferior to men. The struggle had become, rather, one between those who supported the idea that women were capable of occupying the same position in society as men – in the way that one penny can be fitted exactly over another – and those who, whilst recognising their importance, considered their role should be different from that played by men.

On the subject of intellect, however, The Age we Live In seemed to see not an improvement but a deterioration. In the following dialogue the familiar little group were reviewing, in disguised terms, the current issues of their contemporaries:

'Palpable intellect *even now*', said my aunt, pausing with a sigh as though looking down the years that were gone and appraising the difference of vitality in interest with their passing, 'exercises an almost mesmeric influence over me'. 'Intellectual people are very scarce', said Ernestine, 'And people who make you feel its presence by their conversation still rarer', said Julia. 'The two gifts are not always united', I remarked.[22]

This had not been the language of the *Owlet Papers* in 1861 – seven years earlier.

Woman's World laid very little emphasis on dress. It published a monthly two-page supplement on the Paris fashions and, on the whole, left it at that. In May 1868 it did, however, notice that the crinoline had gone out – but expected it soon to return. In June, The Age we Live In opened with the question:

'Well John, what news? . . . Now do not keep me waiting, I hate suspense.'
'But people differ so much in their definition of news, with some it means that all-important question of long or short skirts.'
'Call them by their proper names, John, *robe à la queue* and *robe courte*.'
'Well I read in the *Pall Mall Gazette* a few days ago that the battle of skirts was raging fiercely in Paris.'[23]

And so the onus for this discussion of the frivolities of dress was put on the masculine *Pall Mall Gazette*, the favourite target.

In the following month, July, the monthly supplement of *Woman's World* declared that the 'Watteau toilettes gain ground daily in Paris'.[24] The crinoline had gone for good, a fact that *The Owl* had noticed three months previously:

The reign of the crinoline has passed, and the ample dress subsided into a long tail. This tail was too monstrously inconvenient. It not only draggled and swept up dust, but it gathered round the limbs of persons distant from the wearer, and the question arose as to how to get rid of it. Common sense suggested 'cut it off', but capricious Fashion has put into the head of Beauty the notion of hitching it up.[25]

The Owl, like *Punch* which it rather resembled, was one of the high-class journals to show a mild support for the idea that women were badly treated, a popular topic of the day even outside the pages of women's magazines. Although it had not supported John Stuart Mill on the subject of the enfranchisement of women *Owl* saw that in many fields their lot could, quite harmlessly, be improved. As early as 1864, for instance, after a debate in the Commons, it had printed a 'Cry from the Ladies Gallery' by a Modern Lovelace:

When Stella, dressed for better things
 Enters the 'Commons' Gates,
And her divinest glances brings
 To listen at the grates,
She sweeps the bars with tangled hair
 Imploring with the eye—
Like some poor bird that longs the air
 And wants its liberty.

  . . . .

'Oh why do they this prison make,
 And why this latticed cage,
As though the eyes they cause to ache
 Have danger for their age?
The Peers' high dome a sight affords
 Of far more gallantry,
For ladies in the House of Lords
 Enjoy their liberty.

Of luring them from work the right
 They fear that beauty claims,
I'd sooner try to set alight
 The circumambient Thames.
Then ever from our gallery
 We'll breathe the still small cry—
To gaze and gazed upon to be
 Give us full liberty.'[26]

In breathing her still small cry *The Owl's* Stella undertook, at the same time, not to attempt to set the Thames on fire; the liberties that could safely be demanded were minor and few. Indeed, in December 1868 *Woman's World* itself evidently felt compelled to modify its policy. It had, in any case, received nasty comments from its contemporaries after ascribing, in its previous issue, a very well-known line of Wordsworth's to Byron.[27] Now it announced its decision to rename itself *Kettledrum* (the current word for social gatherings round the tea-table) and to confine itself to tea-table topics. Not that it would impose an absolute ban on articles on women's rights, for it would always be prepared to publish both sides of the question. The aim was clearly to please everyone for while admitting that 'there is a line beyond which feminine minds and feminine pens must not venture', *Kettledrum* hoped 'to meet the approval of a numerous class of thinkers'.[28]

The change-over must have been humiliating, but *Kettledrum* managed to retain from *Woman's World* a recent feature, a weekly article by Our Special Butterfly (supposed, presumably, to be a pretty harmless fluttering creature), who managed very occasionally to squeeze in a coy plea for some special concession or some small liberty for women. *Woman's World* had spoken very gently in its last number: 'If I had to head a deputation of ladies to the House of Lords', wrote Butterfly, following an article in the previous week's *Saturday Review* headed Grim Female,

> no cropped heads or strong-minded-looking black dresses for me. . . . 'Electors such as these,' they would say with true masculine discrimination, 'Well-gloved, becomingly bonnetted, and softly-spoken – such electors would surely exercise their right with feminine good sense.' [29]

Kettledrum – it was a weekly like *Woman's World* – called itself a Magazine of Art, Literature and Social Improvement, and published fairly frequent articles on religious matters, a subject *Woman's World* had deliberately avoided. It also included art criticism and reviewed, in a piece headed Picture Parables, Holman Hunt's new painting, *The Awakening Conscience* which certainly dealt with a subject that called for social improvement.[30] *Kettledrum* also kept together the little circle which made up the members of The Age we Live In but gave Dr Caustic a greatly enlarged part. In a conversation which appeared in an early number of *Kettledrum*:

'The Princess Louise has been to call on Miss Garrett,' said Ernestine.

'The darling', exclaimed Julia, 'I call that royal courage; for there is no denying it – the popular tide runs strongly against the woman worker'.[31]

The tide ran so strongly, indeed, that by the end of the year 1869, when *Kettledrum* had existed for only twelve months, it was itself forced to melt into a journal called *Now-a-Days* which promised to include features on events of interest to women, especially those taking place abroad.

Apart from Special Butterfly's reference to becomingly bonneted women, *Kettledrum* had published nothing on fashion, nor had *Woman's World* ever advocated, in its fashion-supplement, either artistic or healthy dress for women. References to Mrs Bloomer and her attitude to dress would have been impossible, for the lapse of time since her advocacy of dress-reforms was long enough to engender ridicule but too short to generate respect, or even interest.

The year of *Kettledrum* saw the publication of *The Subjection of Women* by John Stuart Mill:

It is but of yesterday that women have either been qualified by literary accomplishments or permitted by society, to tell anything to the general public. As yet very few of them dare tell anything, which men, on whom their literary success depends, are unwilling to hear ... The greater part of what women write about women is mere sycophancy to men ... Many ... overstep the mark and inculcate a servility beyond what is desired or relished by any man except the very vulgarest ... This will be less and less the case, but it will remain true to a great extent, as long as social institutions do not admit the same free development of originality in women which is possible to men.[32]

Which might have been written as an obituary of *Woman's World*.

However doughty as a champion, Mill was not, apparently, quite the type of hero to haunt the dreams of women who yearned for equality with men. In the summer of 1868, using as an excuse an exhibition of classical and renaissance sculpture, The Age we Live In had talked of Mill:

> 'Do you know Donatello's St George? There is a fine cast of it at the Crystal Palace; it is my beau ideal of a knightly face . . . If we could but have a knight',
> 'You have Mill',
> 'Yes but—'
> 'But what? You are hard to please today',
> 'Well I want a knight who believes in woman's goodness as well as women's intellect. I do not mean that Mr Mill does not do it, but I want men to believe in us more.'[33]

John Stuart Mill may have been the champion of women but he was not, it seems, their St George.

Woman's World and *Kettledrum* had found nothing to say on the subject of dress reform in the sense in which it had occupied the minds of Mrs Bloomer and her followers and Charles Reade. Both journals had probably avoided the subject deliberately as one which would have been liable to label them as even more eccentric than they already appeared. Meanwhile, nevertheless, members of the medical profession had for several decades been urging both men and women to adopt healthier forms of dress, though none of them had envisaged anything so extreme as the Bloomer. Dr Andrew Combe's famous *Principles of Physiology applied to the preservation of Health and to the development of physical Education,* which was first published in Edinburgh as early as 1834 had reached its fourteenth edition in 1852, when Mrs Bloomer was actually wearing her characteristic dress. Dr Combe's weighty publication was a book on which many later works were based and from which successive authors not only borrowed principles but quoted whole passages without acknowledgement. It laid particular stress on the condition of the skin and on the importance of maintaining the body at the correct temperature. After discussing the heating and airing of rooms, Dr Combe observed:

> Female dress errs in one important particular, even when unexceptional in material and quality. From the tightness

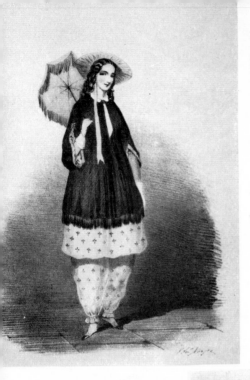

1. Mrs Colonel Bloomer. Cover of a Song-sheet. This is manifestly a music-hall version of Mrs Bloomer, but it represents her in one type of Bloomer costume

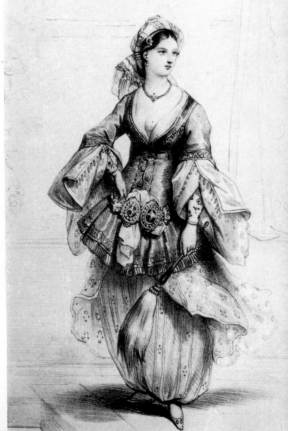

2. Femme Turque. From *Nouveaux Travestissements No. 9*, after an original by Achille Devéria

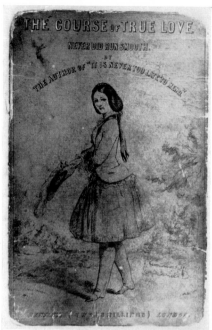

3. Caroline Courtney in her Bloomer – the heroine of *The Course of True Love never did run Smooth* by Charles Reade: 1857. Cover design

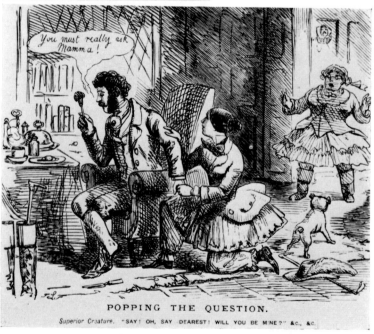

4. One of the delights of Bloomerism – ladies will pop the question. John Leech. *Punch* 1851.

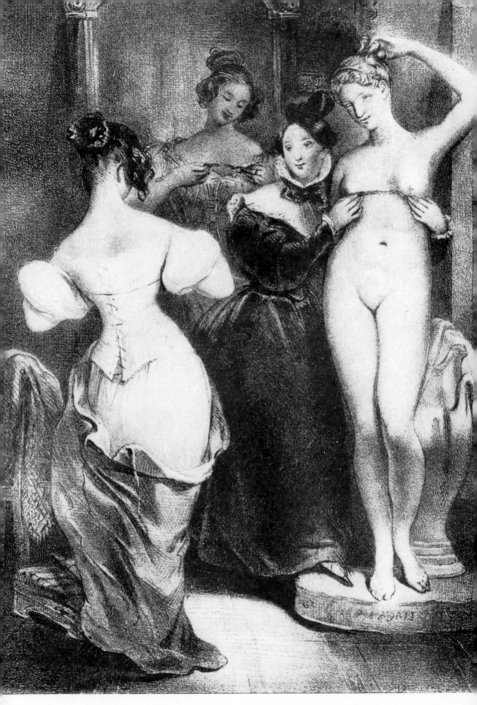

5. Candidates for employment as model in a dressmaker's salon. An important measurement was the width between the breasts; the Venus was not regarded as a standard for the size of the waist. Lithograph by Antoine or Nicolas Maurin. Paris, 1830

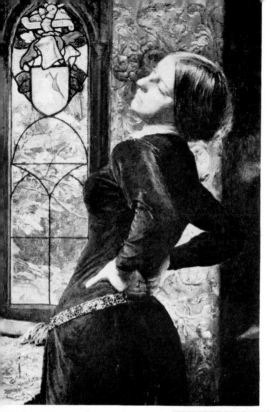

6. 'Mariana', detail, 1851. Sir John E. Millais. The Makins Collection. Ruskin said of this painting that nothing so earnest and complete as the studies of draperies and details had been achieved in art since the days of Albert Dürer.

7. Elizabeth Siddal, 1854. D. G. Rossetti. Cambridge, Fitzwilliam Museum. One of many drawings of Miss Siddal wearing this dress. Here, because her arm is lifted, the loose fit of her bodice can be clearly seen.

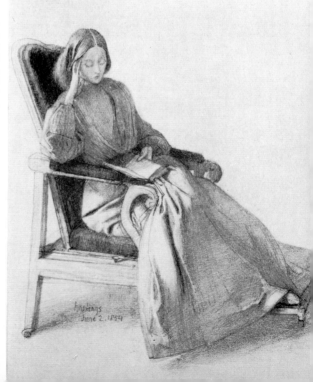

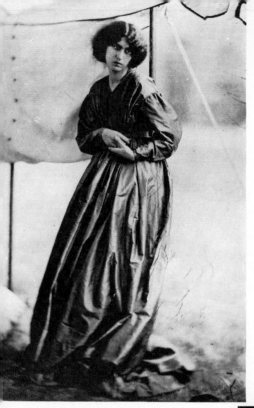

8. Photograph of Jane Morris, posed by Rossetti, 1865. One of several photographs of Mrs Morris wearing a dress with a dropped shoulder-line and a loose back which removes the discomfort otherwise caused by a sleeve set so low down. Gernsheim Collection, University of Texas

9. Mrs Nassau Senior, 1857–8. G. F. Watts. National Trust (Wightwick Manor). Early example of a dress, artistic rather than strictly fashionable, worn by a cultivated woman. Mrs Nassau Senior, a great friend of Watts and of the Rossettis, was a sister of Thomas Hughes of *Tom Brown's Schooldays* fame. She became, in 1874, an Inspector of Workhouses and was closely associated with the movement for Women's Rights

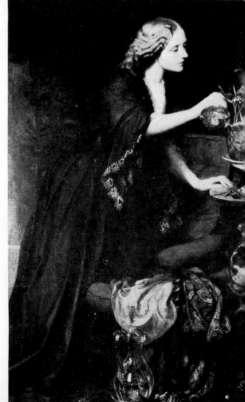

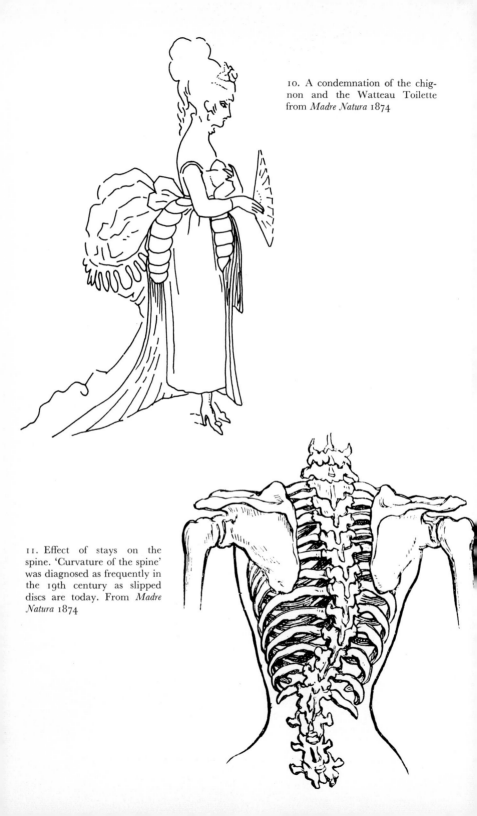

10. A condemnation of the chignon and the Watteau Toilette from *Madre Natura* 1874

11. Effect of stays on the spine. 'Curvature of the spine' was diagnosed as frequently in the 19th century as slipped discs are today. From *Madre Natura* 1874

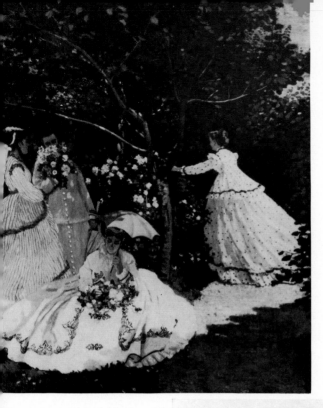

12. 'Femmes au Jardin'. detail, 1867. Claude Monet. Paris, Jeu de Paume. The late crinoline period, when trimmings and colour-contrasts were much bolder than anything worn in the 1850s

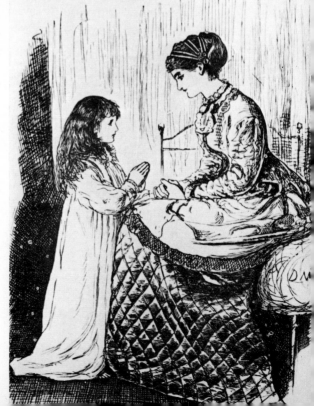

13. The Force of Example. George du Maurier. *Punch* 1873. Grecian bend'lets in the early '70s. 'Now Jessie, say your prayers like a good little girl!' 'Mamma, dear! Why mayn't I kneel down, and hold my *tongue*, as papa does?'

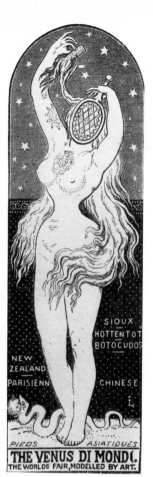

14. The Venus di Mondo. '... impeded respiration and crippled locomotion.' From *Madre Natura* 1874

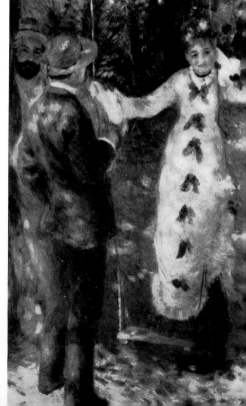

15. 'La Balancoire', detail 1876. Pierre Auguste Renoir. Paris, Jeu de Paume. The long 'princess' line, fashionable between the disappearance of the original crinolette of the early '70s, and the appearance of the new crinolette in the early '80s

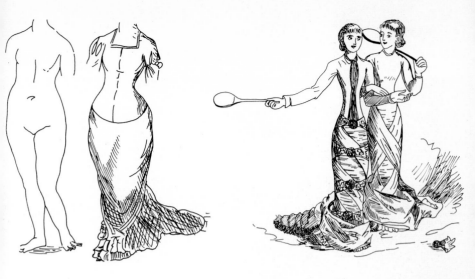

16. (above left) Following the lines of the figure, an apparently 'natural' fashion in dress in which it was difficult to move. From *The Art of Dress* by Mrs Haweis, 1878

17. Live Mummies from *The Art of Dress*. Regarded by Mrs Haweis as over-elaborate versions of the 'princess' line

18. 'The Birth of Venus', detail. Sandro Botticelli. Florence, Uffizi

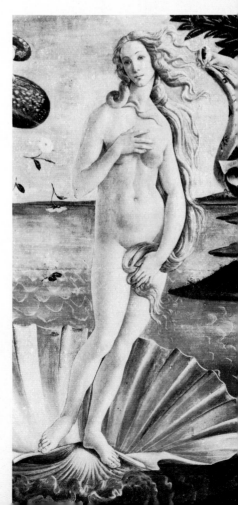

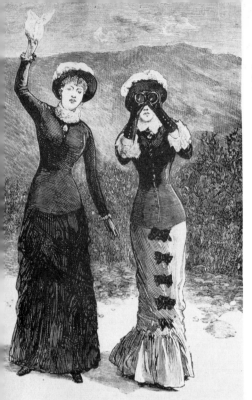

19. 'How Provoking! They Don't See Us.'
The Graphic 1884. On shore in Jamaica. A
somewhat out-of-date version of the long
straight line of the late 1870s can be seen on
the right

20. Woman standing in pose reminiscent of
Botticelli's Venus and wearing 'artistic'
dress. Detail of illustration in *The Pipes of
Pan*, early 1880s, Walter Crane

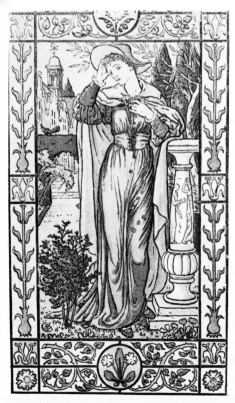

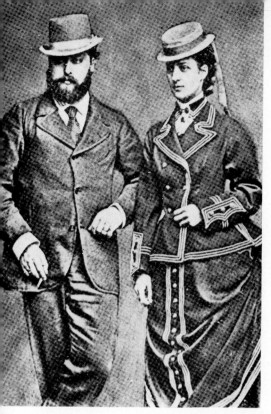

21. Photograph of the Prince and Princess of Wales in 1874. The Princess wears a feminine version of male nautical dress

22. 'Highland Shelter'. Sir John Millais. Private Collection. Effie Ruskin wearing what she called 'a nice jacket', in 1853. Mary Lutyens writes: 'the dress is of brown rough "Linsey Wolsey" which Effie made herself. The tie at the neck is green and belongs to the dress. The jacket is also brown and she is wearing a brown "wideawake" hat'

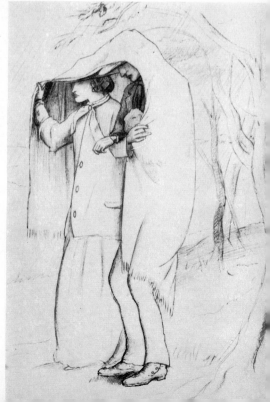

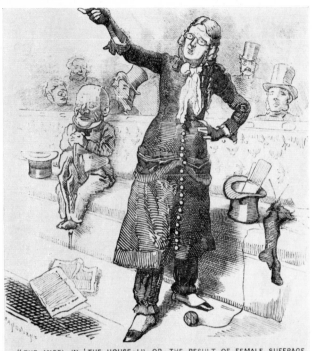

"THE ANGEL IN 'THE HOUSE;'" OR, THE RESULT OF FEMALE SUFFRAGE.
(A Troubled Dream of the Future.)

23. A Bill for the Enfranchisement of women was again presented in the House of Commons in June 1884. *Punch* shows a 'strong-minded woman' wearing a compromise between Bloomer costume and the fashion of 1884. Drawn by Sambourne

24. Mysteries of Heredity. George du Maurier. *Punch* 1888. A late version of the 'strong-minded woman' (in the frogged coat)

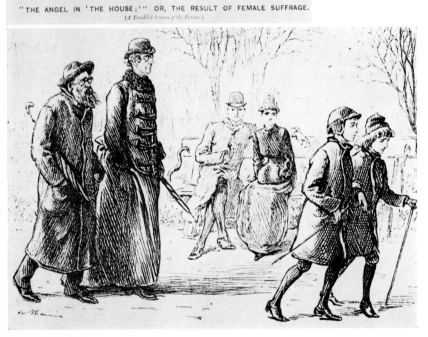

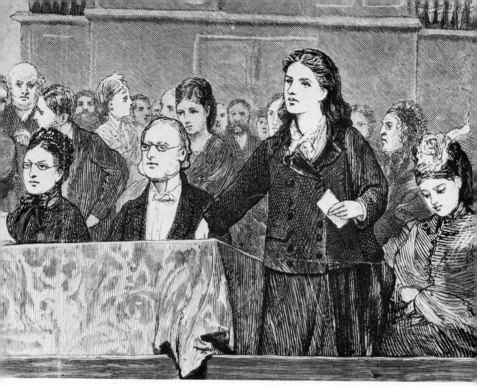

25. Meeting in the Hanover rooms, 1874. Rhoda Garrett, artist cousin of Millicent Fawcett, is speaking. Seated beside her, at the table, is Henry Fawcett, who was already blind at this time. She is wearing the double-breasted jacket regarded as masculine. *The Graphic*

26. Printed cotton, designed by Walter Crane. The 'artistic' 1877 pair wear Patience costumes; compare the profile lady who precedes with figure 30

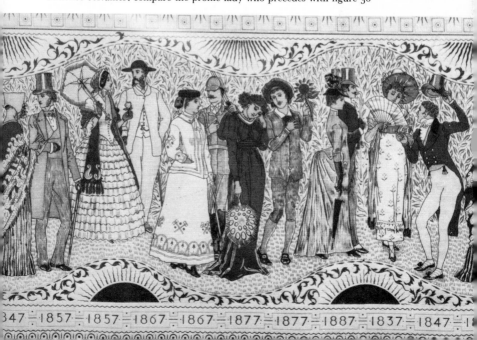

347 ≡ 1857 ≡ 1857 ≡ 1867 ≡ 1867 ≡ 1877 ≡ 1877 ≡ 1887 ≡ 1837 ≡ 1847 ≡ 1

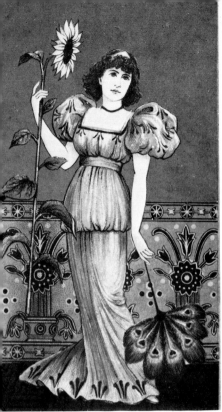

27. Greetings card, early 1880s. Aesthetic dress, probably inspired by *Patience*

28. Passionate Brompton. George du Maurier. *Punch* 1879. The lithe writhing fashion of the end of the '70s and the beginning of the '80s. Says she to him 'are you intense?'

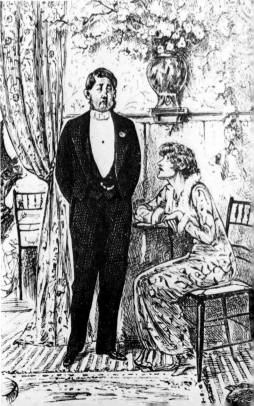

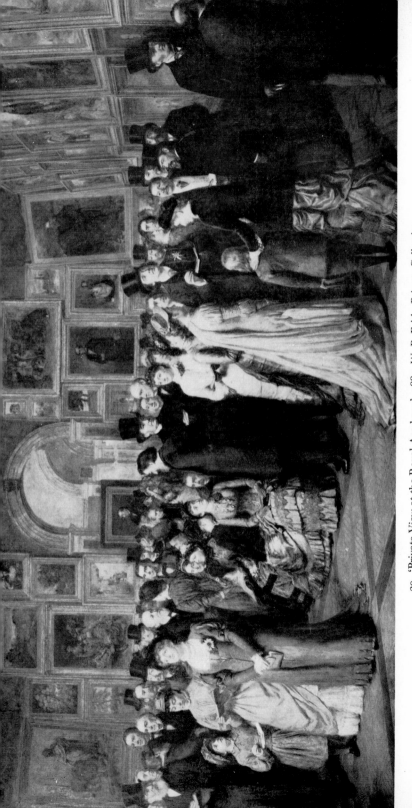

29. 'Private View at the Royal Academy', 1881. W. P. Frith. Private Collection.

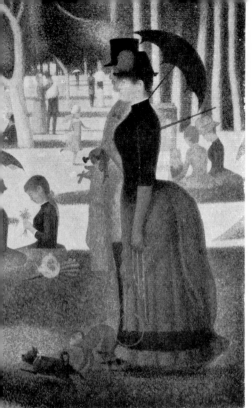

30. 'La Grande Jatte', detail, 1884/5. Georges Seurat. Art Institute of Chicago. 'A waist like a length of pipe': curves disliked by Watts

31. An important consideration. George du Maurier. *Punch* 1884. A fashionable dress with very tight sleeves

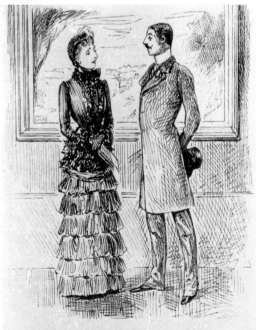

AN IMPORTANT CONSIDERATION.

He. "ARE YOU—A—GOING TO LADY GULPS'S DANCE?"
She. "I—A—DON'T KNOW YET! WHO ASKS HER *MEN* FOR HER?"

with which it is made to fit on the upper part of the body, not only is the insensible perspiration injudiciously and hurtfully confined, but that free play between the dress and the skin, which is so beneficial in gently stimulating the latter by friction at every movement of the body, is altogether prevented, so that the action of the cutaneous nerves and vessels, and consequently the heat generated, are rendered less than what would result from the same dress more loosely worn.[34]

The author then proceeded to warn sportsmen against catching chills and tourists against exposing themselves on mountain tops:

Many of these dangers can be avoided by the wearing of flannel next the skin, for, from its presenting a rough and uneven though soft surface to the skin, every movement of the body in labour or exercise, gives, by consequent friction, a gentle stimulus to the cutaneous vessels and nerves, which assists their actions and maintains their functions in health.[35]

This section of the book includes anecdotes about the experiences of distinguished naval and military commanders who had preserved the health of their men by insisting on the wearing of flannel.

The respect felt for perspiration in the second half of the 19th century was very great and the importance of wearing wool next to the skin was constantly emphasised. A great many books on the healthy life were published, ranging from Dr Combe's 338 pages in double-column small print to popular half-crown hard-backs. Since they usually ran into several editions they must have been read. Most of them included advice on clothing and echoed Dr Combe's principles, and all stressed as he did the menace of cholera and the importance of good ventilation as well as of the daily bath or, at least, the need to wash the whole body all over every day.

The advice did not fall on deaf ears for the attention of the public had been suddenly and violently directed to the dangers of dirt when Florence Nightingale had uncovered a scandal in the hospital at Scutari which sheltered two thousand men suffering from dysentery. During the whole month of November, Miss Nightingale had found, only six shirts had been washed.[36] The incident must have been fresh in the public mind when Charles Reade had caused Caroline Courtney's cook to couple dirt with indecency and it is clear that by this time the connection between dirt and cholera was beginning to be understood by the man in the street.

In the middle years of the 19th century cholera presented a serious danger to the whole of society. There had been a grim outbreak, which had spread widely, in the 1830s and another in the 'forties lingered on until 1855, by which time doctors were seriously disturbed. While it was recognised that the disease was most prevalent in overcrowded working-class areas, authors of medical books also agreed that it was difficult for the poor to find means either to wash or to keep up their strength by wearing wool next to the skin.

Dr Combe himself, in deploring the conditions under which the poor were forced to live, disapproved equally of the risks to health to which women of all classes were exposed. Among the poor he instanced the sempstresses working in fashion houses and remarked that,

Miss —— of Welbeck Street, *an employer*, confesses that in the 'drive of the season' the work is occasionally continued all night *three times a week*.[37]

But, he considered, the health of young girls of the middle classes was also gravely at risk – undermined by the discipline imposed on them. He pointed out that at boarding-schools for young ladies, for instance, the girls were allowed only one daily walk of half an hour as their total exercise and that only in fine weather. He further commented on:

The hurtfulness of the practice in many boarding-schools of sending out girls to walk with a book in their hands, and even obliging them to learn by heart while in the act of walking.[38]

It is significant that unlike contributors to magazines designed to be read by intelligent women, doctors, from their position of strength as respected members of society, could afford to discuss fashions in dress freely and intimately. Dr Combe pointed out:

A ... contrast may be obtained by placing a cast of the Venus de Medicis beside any young woman who, by the diligent employment of stays, has succeeded in converting the form that the Creator bestowed on her, into one which she in her wisdom deems more beautiful ... The statue of the Venus exhibits the natural shape, which is recognised by artists and persons of cultivated taste as the most beautiful which the female figure can assume: accordingly it is aimed at in all the finest statues of ancient and modern times. Misled, however, by ignorance, and a false and most preposterous taste, women of fashion, and their countless flocks of imitators, down even to the lowest ranks of life, have gradually come to regard a narrow or spider-waist as an ornament worthy of attainment at any cost or sacrifice.[39] [5]

In 1829, when Dr Combe had written his first article on the dangers of tight-lacing, an organised movement for the enfranchisement of women was undreamed of. Even in the late 1860s, more than thirty years after Dr Combe's book had first appeared, the *Woman's World* had found itself either too much occupied with matters it considered of greater importance, or too much afraid of losing readers, to advocate a slackening of the stay-laces. The need for a type of dress that was both healthy and not unbeautiful had been seen, therefore, before the middle of the 19th century and by doctors. Stressing utility, but producing something coquettish all the same, Mrs Bloomer was next on the road. The long pause that followed the efforts of these pioneers was mainly filled by personal attempts on the part of the wives of some artists and their patrons to find a dress that was becoming and, at the same time allowed them to move freely. It was not until the 1870s that serious and prolonged attention was given to creating a kind of dress that would combine beauty with a healthy usefulness.

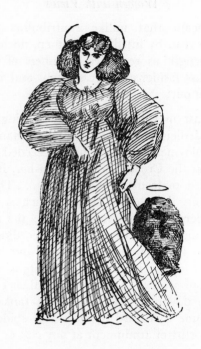

2

PreRaphaelite Clothing

In the late 1840s three young men, two of whom had been
regular students in the Royal Academy and the third an
occasional student, drew up what amounted to a manifesto
incorporating principles, not only of painting but of art in its
widest sense, to which they committed themselves. In 1848,
when the most earnest preliminary discussions on their aims
were taking place, even the label 'PreRaphaelite' was intended
to be a private one, known only to themselves and represented
by the initials PRB (the last for 'Brotherhood') but in the normal
course of things it soon became well known.

John Millais, William Holman Hunt and the immediately

co-opted Dante Gabriel Rossetti, were profoundly opposed to what they regarded as the treacly tide of worn-out academism in which they saw the whole of English painting submerged. As early as the 17th century academies had laid down rules no less insistent than those put forward by the PreRaphaelites, though very different from them; they had suited the classicism of the age that followed and had included instruction in correct composition, disposition and intensity of colour and even on the garments in which characters, especially those of classical antiquity, should be presented. But in 1840 classicism itself was unfashionable in intellectual circles.

The first complaint of the PreRaphaelites was that the current academic practice made the truthful recording of Nature impossible; the second, that art itself was debased by the suavity of treatment and the triviality of the subjects which most artists chose to paint. 'Art's office is not to encourage ... maudlin culture, for true refinement in design, as in word poetry, is to raise aspirations to the healthy and the heroic; it certainly should not lead its admirers to court the moribund, by decking up the sentimentally languid in fine feathers',[1] affirmed Hunt. The rejection of the languid in favour of the healthy would certainly have pleased Dr Combe. 'To those who look upon art as a pretty toy, the earnestness of the notes which were passing through the minds of some of us during this critical time ... may seem out of place as sacred music at a ball',[2] Hunt had continued, as time and time again he underlined the 'resolution of Millais and myself to turn more devotedly to Nature as the one means of purifying art ... painting the whole out of doors, direct on the canvas itself, with every detail I can see, and with the sunlight brightness of the day itself'.[3] In fact, PreRaphaelite principles embodied the 'doctrine of childlike submission to Nature'.[4]

Writing the history of the Brotherhood in his old age, Holman Hunt explained that the PreRaphaelite purpose was to denigrate neither Raphael nor his titanic contemporaries, Michelangelo and Leonardo, but to 'abjure alliance with re-classicalism' –[5] which was seen as the aim of Raphael's immediate imitators and followers, Raphaelites – and to 'avoid revived quattro – or cinque-centism, already powerfully represented in England'.[6]

If the movement in its earliest and purest form was the result of the fleeting dream of three very young men, it was not too ephemeral for its spirit to be caught and transmitted to paper by the sprightly Charles Reade, ever sensitive to the frailest flutter of a new idea. In a totally forgotten novel *Christie Johnstone*, written in 1850 (though, perhaps significantly, not published until 1853), the hero is Charles Gatty, a young and struggling artist who, to a sceptic convinced that no painter can both talk and paint, replies,

> 'Then I'll say but one word more and it is this. The artifice of painting is old enough to die; it is time that the art was born. Whenever it does come into the world, you will see no more dead corpses of trees, grass, water, robbed of their life, the sun-light, and flung upon canvass in a studio by the light of a cigar, and a lie – and ... with these little swords' (waving his brush) 'we'll fight for nature-light, truth-light and sunlight against a world in arms, no, worse, in swaddling clothes'.[7]

The young PreRaphaelites had already found their publicist.

In a period when the English countryside was considerably more accessible than it is today no serious problems, apart from bad weather, were involved in the painting of landscape, and the geological and botanical objects which could form interesting foregrounds, direct from Nature. Animals, human and otherwise, proved more difficult. Assistants had to be employed, for instance, to hold down individual sheep in the positions required by the paintings' implied narratives and Millais was, on one occasion, singularly lucky in accidentally killing a mouse which died in exactly the attitude in which he wanted to paint it. Human beings furthermore, had to be capable of assuming expressions and clothes which were appropriate to the situation as well as to the period intended in the paintings.

The logical outcome of the combination of a childlike submission to nature and a determination to 'choose an educational outflow from a channel where the stream had no pollution of egoism and was innocent of pandering to corrupt thoughts and passions'[8] was that the search for themes through which both these aspects of PreRaphaelitism could be perfectly demonstrated became of the utmost importance. Shakespeare could prove a fruitful source since his essential Englishness meant that even *Two Gentlemen of Verona* could settle comfortably into an English landscape. The clothes in which they could be presented were a different matter.

Sources of information for fashions of the past are three: surviving garments, literary descriptions and contemporary pictorial representations. To painters committed to PreRaphaelite principles, at least the last two of these forms of evidence were clearly unsatisfactory, and even surviving garments (few, if any, from periods that the PreRaphaelites were most tempted to paint) were usually shabby and fragmentary. Millais did buy a 'really splendid lady's ancient dress – all flowered over in silver embroidery'[9] in which to paint Ophelia floating submerged in her stream, but this was a rare find.

Literary references to dress could evoke poetic images; Rossetti, for instance, followed the Song of Solomon, 'She shall be brought unto the King in raiment of needlework' and painted his *Beloved* in an embroidered dress (made from a Japanese kimono), but literature could not provide the actuality which PreRaphaelite painters required. Nor could costume in works of Old Masters be more useful in this respect since absolute fidelity to Nature demanded direct observation of the folds imposed on drapery by the specific poses and actions of their wearers which must, moreover, be seen in the lighting chosen by the painter for his scene. PreRaphaelite painters held strong views as to the behaviour and stance assumed by human beings under emotional stress, an ingredient of most of their pictures;their views often showed a respect for some earlier painters who had undertaken similar scenes, but they certainly did not coincide with them.

The only expedients left to the Brotherhood, therefore, were either to have specially designed clothing made for their sitters to be painted in, or to rely on secondary sources, of

which there were two: books on historical costumes and
current productions of operas or historical dramas (which
could be regarded as tertiary sources since stage costume was
probably derived from costume books). Neither of these alter-
natives proved entirely satisfactory. The first was expensive
since fidelity to what they thought of as natural reconstructions
of their chosen subjects often demanded costly fabrics; costume
books shared with surviving pictorial representations the
disadvantage of showing only one aspect of any one dress and,
in addition, those who wrote them seldom really understood
what the clothes they wrote about had actually been like. The
theatre was a clumsy alternative since the taste of theatrical
designers was unlikely to correspond to that of PreRaphaelite
painters. Millais did go to see Meyerbeer's opera *The Huguenots*,
'to study the pose and the costumes of the actors'[10] when he
was preparing to paint his *Huguenot* picture, but such an
opportunity cannot have occurred often.

Recent research has shown that Ford Madox Brown,
Millais and Rossetti used, with varying degrees of accuracy,
Camille Bonnard's *Costume Historique*, published in Paris in
two volumes in 1829–30.[11] Millais' Isabella, for example, bears a
distant resemblance to his tracing of Beatrice d'Este, redrawn
by Bonnard, or rather his illustrator Paul Mercuri, from the
Pala Sforzesca, but Millais' Isabella is far more like a girl of the
PreRaphaeilite circle than the Duchess of Milan.

Careful study of paintings by the PreRaphaelite group during
the short period of their close relationship shows that they were
certainly able to benefit from seeing each other at work, even
where the dress was concerned. Rossetti, for instance, in his
drawings and water-colours of the *Sanc Grael*, must have been
inspired by the dress which Millais had made for his *Mariana*.
Millais, when he was actually preparing to start on his two
paintings, the *Woodman's Daughter* and *Mariana* wrote to a
friend saying, 'I am deep in the mystery of purchasing velvets
and silk draperies for my pictures. The shopman simpers with
astonishment at the request coming from a male biped'.[12] The
designs of the two velvet garments required in these paintings –
the tunic of the squire's son and the dress of Mariana herself –

were probably provided by Millais' mother who, 'being more gifted than most women', grounded him in history, poetry, literature etc., knowledge of costume and armour, all of which was of the greatest use to him in his career.[13] 'As for mamma, she reads to me and finds me subjects. She gets me all I want in the way of dresses, and makes them up for me, and searches out difficult questions for me at the British Museum'[14] he had told Hunt.

Mariana's blue velvet dress of 14th-century cut made an extremely important contribution to the painting.[6] Each tense velvet fold is not only the result of the pose of the healthy girl chosen by Millais as his model but is expressive of the exasperated frustration experienced by the original girl in Keats' poem. The dress is manifestly painted from an actual model.

Pictorial representations of 14th-century fashions were not difficult to find, but paintings of episodes from the Bible, though cheaper to dress, presented graver problems. The sheep crowding to peer over the wattle-fence into St Joseph's workshop in Millais' *Christ in the House of his Parents*, he was able to paint from two sheep's heads with the wool still on, bought from a local butcher, but where could authentic models for the Holy Family be found? Since every crease and wrinkle of stuff must be painted direct from the actual object set in the correct light and must correspond to the wearer's station in life as well as to the emotion of the moment, everything must actually exist before it could be painted.

To clothe the Virgin who kneels in front of the carpenter's bench, Millais was almost certainly able to use a dress from the wardrobe of a member of his immediate circle of Pre-Raphaelite painters or their friends. Her veil is contrived from a piece of thick linen or cotton, appropriate to a working-class girl but unfunctional in its shape. He had used the same arrangement (and probably the same piece of stuff) to provide a hood for one of the male diners in his painting *Lorenzo and Isabella*, exhibited in 1848 – the previous year. It was the kind of historical lapse that the considerably more rigidly doctrinaire Holman Hunt must have deplored. For the fur loin-cloth of the little John the Baptist, Millais probably resorted to the butcher already referred to; St Joseph's assistant wears his own under-pants rolled up, beneath a drapery made from a piece of cotton from the Middle East.

Such expedients could sometimes serve to furnish the 'truth' on which PreRaphaelite painting so greatly depended; 'beauty' could not, however, be guaranteed to appear by this means. The painful dichotomy which harassed those anxious to produce, later in the century, clothing which could be accepted as both rational and beautiful, was already distressing those members of the public who were first confronted by PreRaphaelitism in the later 1840s.

Rossetti's first PreRaphaelite painting, the *Girlhood of the Virgin Mary* suffered less from the anger of the public than Millais' picture discussed above. His sister Christina sat for the figure of the young Virgin and almost certainly wore, for the painting, a dress from her own wardrobe, very near in style to what was, twenty years later, to be labelled by fashion journalists, PreRaphaelite dress.

In 1848, when Rossetti was painting his *Girlhood of the Virgin*, this pale grey dress, if worn in the street, would have looked affectedly lumpish and only the quietness of its colour and its complete absence of ornament could have saved it from ridicule, if it was so saved. The painting was spared some of the vituperation directed the following year at Holman Hunt and Millais partly, no doubt, because Christina Rossetti looked modest and pretty as the Virgin Mary and her mother comely as St Anne, whose nun-like head draperies, though falsely contrived, escaped the eccentricity of the equally absurd arrangement of the veil worn by Millais' Virgin. For the rest of her clothing Rossetti's St Anne wears a plainly cut bodice of a style fashionable in the 1840s, which fits closely to her corseted figure, and over it a studio-drapery to serve as a cloak. The dress itself was, in all probability, taken from Mrs Rossetti's ward-robe. Since this is a 'costume picture' the fact that Christina wore no petticoats beneath her dress could be accepted; in a drawing-room the sharp outline of her knees would have given offence.

As we know, in the long run neither Millais nor Rossetti was to be happy under the strict discipline of PreRaphaelite principles. Holman Hunt, their true begetter, was alone in insisting that they should govern his whole career. Writing of the search for corners of the English countryside (not too far from London) which could provide appropriate backgrounds for their chosen subjects – Hunt's *Hireling Shepherd* and Millais' *Ophelia* – it was Hunt who spoke of the beauty and perfection of the spot, and Millais of the flies.

Apart from his two paintings, *Two Gentlemen of Verona* and *Claudio and Isabella*, Holman Hunt avoided the problems which arose in trying, with scientific accuracy, to paint dress of a period in the past from which no specimens survived. He was severely censured for clothing his Christ, *The Light of the World*, in a priestly alb and cope, but both of these could be painted from life. The attacks could not have been purely the result of Protestant distaste for the use of vestments, for the cope had become relatively acceptable since the Archbishop of Canterbury had worn one at the coronation of Queen Victoria. Hunt determined, in any case, to go to Palestine where he could paint his scriptural pictures in the places where the events they tell of actually happened.

Less obsessed with verisimilitude than Hunt, it was Rossetti, nevertheless, who recorded the exact form of dress later to be labelled 'PreRaphaelite'. The form of dress, that is to say, which was certainly worn by Elizabeth Siddal and, a little modified to conflict less with the later fashion, by Jane Morris. Its prototype probably belonged as we have seen, to Christina Rossetti; this earlier version may, perhaps, be found in a pen and ink study of 1846 for a *Hermia and Helena* group which Rossetti apparently carried no further.

Fashionable dress of the 1840s, although gentle in outline, was physically restrictive, partly because it was laced very tightly round the ribs, partly because a number of petticoats were necessary to build the skirt out to the required bell-shape, but above all because the sleeve was set, not on to the top of the shoulder but into a line two or three inches below it, on the upper arm. This meant that since the bodice was held firmly down round the waist the arms could only be raised to a very limited extent. This dropped shoulder-seam was still fashionable in the middle of the 1860s.

In drawings of Elizabeth Siddal, done in 1855[15] as studies for his painting of *Dante's vision of Rachel and Leah,* Rossetti made it clear that not only was Miss Siddal not wearing a crinoline (in fashionable dress approaching its widest span at this date) but that the sleeves of her dress were set well up on to the shoulder, thus giving complete freedom of arm movement. Furthermore the front of her bodice is concealed by an arrangement of drapery probably designed to hide the fact that it was not very tightly laced. [7] A very similar dress can be found in a preliminary drawing for the *Sanc Grael,* done from life but evidently before Rossetti had decided on the *Mariana* type of dress for Guinevere. Another drawing, also of Miss Siddal, done probably about the same time but used much later for *Beata Beatrix,* shows Miss Siddal in a very similar dress with the sleeve set fairly high on the shoulder, but no front drapery.

In 1865 William Morris's wife, Jane, was photographed in a pose chosen by Rossetti. [8] By this time the fashionable waist had risen slightly and this is reflected in the placing of Jane Morris's waist-belt which holds in a bodice not tightly laced but draped in front. In this dress the sleeve is set below the shoulder but with some fulness at the shoulder-seam, a characteristic of later dress based on that worn by ladies in the PreRaphaelite circle. In the photograph the back of the dress is hidden, but Rossetti's painting *The Day Dream,* for which Mrs Morris was the sitter, shows clearly that the dress, which she wore for this painting, had a back so full that in spite of the low-placed shoulder-seam the arm would be able to move quite freely. The fact that *The Day Dream* was commissioned in 1879 and is dated 1880, when both sleeves and bodices were fitted extremely tightly to the body, shows that Jane Morris almost certainly continued to wear 'PreRaphaelite' dress which would have looked even more unconventional in 1880 that it must have done in 1865 when she was photographed.

As it happens, a second photograph of Jane Morris wearing

the same dress has survived[16] and from this we can see that it is
not a dress divided into a bodice and skirt at all but is, in fact,
a great bell-shaped Watteau-like affair. with folds falling as
soft pleats from the shoulder at the back. This is a startling
discovery since two or three years later the crinoline suddenly
disappeared and was replaced, temporarily, by what was called
a 'Watteau' gown designed and launched by the Paris *haute
couture*.

Although in the early preparatory drawings for his finished
compositions, Rossetti usually made careful studies of his
models wearing their own dress, in the paintings themselves
(apart from the first two which were dominated by Pre-
Raphaelite principles) he pursued 'beauty' rather than 'truth'
in the PreRaphaelite sense. The sources of the ingredients
in his exquisitely *haute cuisine* are fascinating to explore but
this is not the place to do it.

In Holman Hunt's opinion Rossetti's water-colours (now
amongst his most admired works) often lapsed into a second-
hand mediaevalism which was totally alien to PreRaphaelite
taste. Rossetti did not share Hunt's refusal to depend on earlier
works of art for costumes and furnishings in his paintings; on
the contrary, not only did he use tomb-sculptures and manu-
script paintings as sources for costumes but he also used over
and over again, whatever the ostensible period or subject of his
painting, any piece of brocade or contrived head-dress – con-
structed probably by himself in the first place – if it appealed
to his sense of beauty. An extraordinary bag-like hood, pinned-
up, no doubt, on the spur of the moment and worn by Fanny
Cornforth gathering apples, he used in at least three drawings
or water-colours on vaguely 'mediaeval' themes.[17]

In the earliest years of discussions between the three original
members of the PRB, Holman Hunt recorded that on the
occasion of his first visit to him, Rossetti had deplored the base
and vulgar forms and incoherent curves in contemporary
furniture and, Hunt continues, 'we speculated on improvement
in all household objects, furniture, fabrics, and other interior
decorations. Nor did we pause till Rossetti enlarged upon the
devising of ladies' dresses and the improvement of man's

costume, determining to follow the example of early artists not in one branch of taste only, but in all.'[18]

It is impossible to estimate the extent to which Rossetti's personal inventions influenced the clothes worn by his women friends and his friends' wives. That he showed a feeling for developments in contemporary fashion is demonstrated by a portrait of Mrs F. R. Leyland called *Monna Rosa*, painted in 1867 when the crinoline was rapidly disappearing from fashion. Rossetti painted Mrs Leyland draped in a piece of 18th-century brocade which can be found in several of his pictures and which evidently belonged to him. It is significant that the lines of the tucked-in and pinned-together stuff in which Mrs Leyland is draped foreshadow exactly the composition which was to replace the crinoline.

The circle of women who actually wore PreRaphaelite dress during the period of the Brotherhood's existence was not confined to Rossetti's models – Elizabeth Siddal, Fanny Cornforth and Jane Morris – for Effie Ruskin on holiday in the Highlands in the 1860s appears in sketches by Millais wearing picturesquely comfortable clothing which closely resembles it, [22] while Mrs Nassau Senior who, according to Millais' son, was the model for the mother in Millais' *Rescue*, was painted in her own character by Watts wearing an embroidered dress which, if not actually PreRaphaelite, was certainly 'artistic'. [9]

Looking back from the end of the 19th century and writing in the journal *Aglaia* in the autumn of 1894, Walter Crane had this to say about the influence of the PreRaphaelites on the design of women's dress,

I think there can be no doubt ... of the influence in our time of what is commonly known as the PreRaphaelistic school and its later representatives in this direction ... But it is an influence which never owed anything to academic teaching. Under the new impulse, the new inspiration from the mid-century from the purer and simpler lines, forms and colours of early mediaeval art, the dress of women in our own time may be seen to have been transformed for a while, and, though the pendulum of fashion swings to and fro, it does not much affect, except in small details, a distinct type of dress which has become associated with artistic people – those who seriously study and consider of the highest value and importance beautiful and harmonious surroundings in daily life. . . . Beginning in the households of the artists themselves, the type of dress to which I allude, by imitation . . . soon became spread abroad until in the seventies and early eighties we saw the fashionable world and the stage aping, with more or less grotesque vulgarity, what it was fain to think were the fashions of the inner and most refined artistic cult.[19]

The article in which this passage appeared was one of four, under the general title, *On the Progress of Taste in Dress*; Walter Crane's contribution was sub-titled, *In relation to Art Education*. By that time PreRaphaelite painting had passed into art history but forty years earlier, in 1853, when Charles Reade's *Christie Johnstone* was published, Reade had felt it necessary to explain in a tail-piece that although 'one or two topics are not treated exactly as they would be if written . . . today' he wanted, nevertheless, to 'lay at the feet of the public a faulty but genuine piece of work, and a truth that was struggling for bare life in the year of truth 1850',[20] which seems to suggest that by 1853 the struggle had already become less intense.

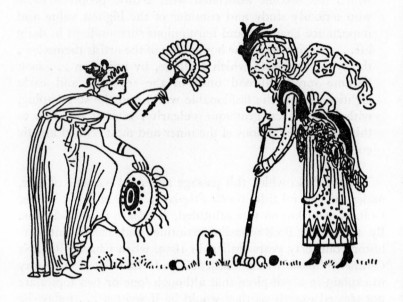

3

Grecian Fillets

At the time of its demise in 1868, the crinoline was thought of as ugly. Its rapid and complete disappearance was a sign that it had lasted too long and outlived its period. Its replacement, very temporarily, by a straight skirt with a long train, and then almost immediately by what *Woman's World* and others quite irrationally called the 'Watteau toilette', involved one of those major changes of fashion that produce a new aesthetic composition and which demand, in consequence, a change in the behaviour of the wearer.

The dome-shaped skirt of the 1840s, enlarged in the 'fifties by a crinoline sub-structure, because it was symmetrical, had looked the same from whatever side it was viewed. By the middle of the 'sixties this all-round appearance was modified a little by a slight extension at the back, but this did not really make much difference. Manufacturers of the various supports designed to hold out the skirt did their best to give some variety to a basic shape that had become a bore. For instance, just before the crinoline's disappearance the 'Ondine', made in large flutes, was intended, as its name implies, to produce in the skirt a gracefully wavy effect, and the same firm's 'Ebonite', composed of light and very flexible india-rubber hoops, was advertised, like the 'Ondine' not only in women's magazines but also in the masculine *Owl*.[1] Both the undulating shape and the extreme flexibility were certainly aimed at destroying the uncompromisingly stable appearance of the basic dome, in the centre of which each female wearer was unapproachably planted.

The sudden jettisoning of this symmetrical design for one of complete asymmetry was dramatic. In contrast to the crinoline, the new fashion possessed, for instance, a 'most favourable viewpoint'; for while the frontal elevation of the 'Watteau toilette' had little character to commend it, its side elevation was very striking indeed. Corresponding to the bunched-up puff of fabric which swelled out below the waist at the back – held and emphasised by bows of ribbon with fluttering ends – the hair was drawn away from the face and massed at the back of the head to produce what was named a 'chignon', formed of huge, loose, intertwined plaits or rolling curls. [10]

Seen from the side the wearer seemed to press forward, followed by her trappings: to be transformed into an unctuous version of the winged Victory of Samothrace – a resemblance of which she may have been vaguely conscious. For the arrival of the new fashion was soon followed by a new deportment – a thrusting forward of the breasts and backward of the buttocks – termed the 'Grecian bend'. The new fashion also coincided with a craze for the new sport of roller-skating, in the practice of which it showed at its best. Flying round the skating-rink, curls and draperies were blown violently backwards while the torso, firmly encased in a close-fitting mould, looked as brave and compact as the prow of a ship.

This change in composition was radical and unexpected; changes in fashionable colour-schemes, though they emerged more slowly, were no less fundamental. The rococo combinations of, for example, rose-pink with pea-green, or lilac with pale chrome-yellow, which make the dress of the 1850s appear in retrospect one of the 'prettiest' in history, were replaced in the 'sixties by far more sullen effects. During this decade dome-shaped skirts of thick pewter-grey silk were cut horizontally by a wide band of black velvet, and black ornamentation was, in fact, very popular. In strongly defined borders and bands composed, often, of thick fringes with intermittent hanging tassels, black was used to decorate a new colour of the period – 'electric' blue, a harsh and slightly greenish thunderous shade. By the middle of the 1860s only dresses designed for high summer were allowed to retain the airiness of the 'fifties and even these, as can be seen, for instance, in Monet's *Femmes au Jardin*, [12] were punctuated by accents of colour in contrasts stronger in tone than would have been permissible during the ten previous years.

Those who see in the design of clothes a reflection of at least some aspects of the society which produces it, would be justified in regarding the transformations of the late 1860s as vindicating their theory. From the point of view of composition women could be thought of as having stepped out of the encircling bird-cage to assume a forward-looking attitude well suited to their sociological and educational aspirations, while, at the same time, the insipid charm of earlier colour-schemes was replaced by effects which if not actually violent were certainly aggressive.

This was not, however, at all the way that the crinoline and the Watteau toilette looked to those who actually saw them being worn, for both were thought of as ugly. Charles Reade had described the skirt of Elizabeth I as a 'bloated bell' which was 'imitated by her successor in New York' and the Watteau toilette was alleged by later commentators to make women look deformed. At the beginning of the 1870s, by which time the Watteau toilette had been generally adopted, it was not only artists and their friends but many others too who began consciously to long for the abolition of fashion altogether in favour of something permanent, something which, because it combined beauty with utility, need never be changed. Among these were women who naturally looked for reform in other directions too.

The craving seems to have been officially expressed first at a congress of the Council of German women held in Stuttgart in 1868 and reported in the final number of *Woman's World*. It was the second congress of the Council, which included in its aims the establishment of a chain of 'Women's Museums' where lectures on those subjects presided over by the Muses could be held. The Stuttgart congress of 1868 (the year of the abandonment of the crinoline in favour of the Watteau toilette) put forward a Motion for a 'reform in dress' after a discussion on 'ways and means' of resisting the 'tyranny and vagaries of fashion'.

The Stuttgart Motion was prophetic of ideals that were to be cherished both in Germany and in England over the following two decades; its terms were:

(*a*) That nothing that has already proved to be beautiful and convenient, to be declared old-fashioned or out-of-date.

(*b*) Nothing to be adopted that does not meet demands of taste and suitability.

(*c*) To hold aloof from garments and articles of toilet that are injurious to health, and that women should adopt a style of dress in accordance with their husbands' and fathers' incomes.[3]

This was not the first time that suggestions for a reform of women's dress had appeared in Germany: at the end of the 18th century, Daniel Chodowieki, a Danziger working in Berlin, had designed rather lumpy versions of the neo-classic garments that were about to make their way into the current fashion. Since, however, Chodowieki's reforms were overtaken by fashion itself, his designs are mainly interesting as reflections of the concern expressed by his contemporary German philosophers on the subject of aesthetic morality. Earlier in his career Chodowieki had produced a pair of engravings contrasting 'sincere' with 'artificial' sentiment. Both portray a man and a woman admiring a sunset: the sincere couple gaze upon it with sober reverence whereas those whose sentiment is artificial greet it with baroque gestures of appreciation. By this standard Chodowieki's reformed dress belonged to a category 'sincere' – that is to say it was plain in outline and almost without ornamentation.

Chodowieki's reformed dress had soon been eclipsed by the similar though much more glamorous fashions launched in the Paris drawing-rooms inhabited by the new beauties who emerged with the Directoire and the early days of Napoleon's rule. It had certainly long been forgotten, except perhaps by historians of dress, by the time the Council of German women arrived, by a different route, at the idea that changes of fashion were, somehow, unworthy. And it was this attitude that must surely have accounted for the omission of a fashion-supplement from the otherwise docile *Kettledrum* which had promised to limit itself to 'tea-table' themes. With this small gesture of protest it must have attempted to establish the right of women to ignore, if they wished, topics that were thought of as exclusively feminine.

There was, and had been throughout the 19th century, no shortage of magazines devoted to fashion and domestic subjects in a conventional style. Conventional from the point of view of content, that is to say, for in presentation a great change had taken place since the 1860s. The earlier form of magazine, small in page-size and usually illustrated by charmingly delicate engravings (those of fashionable dresses were usually in colour and coloured, of course, by hand), disappeared during the 'sixties and were replaced by journals with bigger pages, lower quality paper, and less refined engravings. These were obviously designed for a less aristocratic public which included those able to buy, order, or make for themselves clothes stitched by machine. Both the sewing-machine, which was invented in the 1850s but not mass-produced until the 'sixties, and the new cheap fashion-papers had sociological implications. Although they would not be entirely acceptable socially for several decades, the invasion of the fashionable world by people of the middle class who depended less on birth and wealth than on ability, was beginning.

With the radical change in the design of fashionable dress at the end of the 'sixties a new kind of beauty began to be admired. The small frail girls with feet no bigger than mice – the young heroines of novels by Dickens – were no longer in favour with artists or in fiction. When Mrs Oliphant published her novel, *At his Gates* in 1872, the fashion was too new for her to adopt it for her actual heroine, but Clara, the foil, spoilt daughter of the plutocrat villain, had the looks of the moment. At eighteen,

> she was a full-blown Rubens beauty, of the class that has superseded the gentler, pensive, unobtrusive heroine in these days.[4]

This was the woman already adopted as a model by Watts and Leighton and Poynter and soon to be painted by Albert Moore in compositions based on the Parthenon frieze. She was indeed Greek in inspiration, for the Venuses so much admired by artists and doctors of medicine were beginning to attract a wider public – the names of Phidias and Praxiteles were becoming familiar enough to be useful to any journalist. In 1868 Matthew Arnold had reviewed, for the *Pall Mall Gazette*, the translation of the first volume of the *History of Greece* by Ernst Curtius, as he was to write about the successive volumes in the following eight years, and from the beginning of the 1870s throughout the next three decades less distinguished writers were repeatedly to call upon the art of the ancient Greeks to support their aesthetic and their sanitary theories.

For aesthetics and health, which to a mild extent had been linked by Dr Combe and his followers were in the 1870s often to be found in each other's company; this meant that the subject of dress was no longer confined to the drawing-rooms of conventional women. Since men now discussed dress, clever

women were no longer compelled to avoid it. In 1868 the
Council of German Women had already associated beauty and
convenience in their demands for a reform in dress; in England
it was not women but men who first called attention both to
the dangers to health of contemporary fashions and to their
lack of resemblance to the clothing of the Greeks.

In 1874 appeared the fourth edition of a decorative little
book first published earlier that year with the title, *Madre
Natura versus the Moloch of Fashion, a social essay*; its author
called himself 'Luke Limner Esq' and dedicated his work to
'John Marshall Esq FRS etc etc, Professor of Surgery, and Art
Anatomy to the Royal Academy and to the Department of
Science and Art'.

The presence in the title of the *Moloch of Fashion* is not
particularly surprising, for Moloch (presumably thought of as a
deity who fed upon the innocent) was constantly required at this
period to represent all that was evil in contemporary life, such
as overcrowding in cities and industrial greed. It could almost
be said to be unusual to discover an article on sociological
problems in which his name did not crop up. His appearance
as the evil supporter of fashion, therefore, must have had the
effect of enhancing its status as a topic.

A coat-of-arms appearing on the title-page of *Madre Natura*
is described within:

The Mantua-Makers' Arms.
On a shield *sable*, a Corset *proper*; crest upon a wreath of
roses and Hour-glass *or*, typical of golden hours wasted.
Supporters, Harpies: the dexter 'Fashion' crowned with a
chignon *or*, corsetted and crinoletted *proper*, her train being
decorated with bows, and the wings with scissors; the
sinister, 'Vanity', crowned with a coronet of pearls and
strawberry leaves bears the wings of a papillon, eyed *proper*,
the queue a la Paon. Motto, 'Fashion unto Death!' [See
title-page]

The motto reads, in fact, *A la Mode à la Mort*. The author
begins with a particularly severe reproof, to the crinoline, a

fashion but lately laid aside which disqualified those who
wore it from the performance of their duties to society, in a
more summary and terrible manner than any perversion of
clothing yet devised by the milliner for the ever-ready
dupes of her specious handicraft. We allude to the victims
destroyed by wearing hoops and crinoline. There are many
who escaped death, who to this day bear evidence of the
sad custom of using aids to distend the dress, carrying
terrible brands, in the form of scars, where the flesh has been
seared, and contracted joints where bones have been broken,
derangements of the system by which chronic aches and
pains are continued to the end of existence.[5] [11]

The small compressed waist which resulted from the tight-
lacing of the corset is next attacked, as

> reversing all the type-harmonies of form and graceful fitness
> of the woman's structure ... We make bold to assert that
> Praxiteles would have deemed her hideously unworthy of
> reproduction by his chisel and her statue by his masterly
> hand would never have graced the Temple of Delphi.[6] [14]

The author then embarked on his main theme:

> But from a point of view more grave, were it even possible –
> which it is not – to disconnect the intimate accordance of the
> aesthetical form from its connate hygienic design throughout
> the whole structure of the human body, we consider the
> subject is one which, if thought convenient for a theme
> likely to be a 'taking one' as 'a question of the day' should
> at least have been treated more in regard to real interests of
> society than in the specious and flippantly sophistic style
> defined by Logicians as the *Argumentum ad Ignorantiam* ...[7]

but the sentence is very long and by no means ends there.
Apart from the connection which the author saw between
'aesthetical form' and 'hygienic design' his reference to the
possibility of the whole thing becoming a 'question of the day'
is significant, for both here and in contemporary novels there

is a suggestion that ideas were on the move and among them appeared a new conception of the essential character of women. In the pages of *Madre Natura* a new sort of woman made her début. This was the 'Girl of the Period' who was to be referred to under that label repeatedly both in sociological studies and in fiction during the two following decades.[8]

Although in the 1870s it was still absolutely necessary for women, whether married or single, to guard their reputations with extreme care, it was evidently becoming possible for a young woman of the middle class to walk in the garden or to spend half an hour in a sitting-room alone with a young man without risking her good name, and elderly gossips who condemned such behaviour could now be ridiculed with impunity. In other words, the rigid code of the 18th century, which was still obeyed in the middle of the 19th, was beginning to be questioned.

'Luke Limner's' championship of *Madre Natura* is written in a colloquial style but its intention is certainly serious. Into a long list of eighteenth century medical authors – most of them Continental – who had published condemnations of physically harmful fashions in dress he inserted the names of philosophers and writers on aesthetics who had been equally critical of the fashions of their day, among them Buffon, Schlegel, Hogarth and Burke.[9] He quoted Vaughan's *Essay Philosophical and Medical, concerning modern clothing*, which had appeared in 1792, in considerable and blood-curdling detail and included Vaughan's view that 'the fault is more in men than in women' for admiring the wearers of harmful fashions.

Following two drawings of female skeletons distorted by the wearing of tight stays, the author of *Madre Natura* placed another which had retained the natural form, saying:

Having indicated the influence of compression upon the interior-organs, we now show its workings with the bony structure, and the terrible effect it exercises upon the lower ribs and spine – the lines of the contracted skeletons contrasting sadly with that of the beautiful Venus de Medici, represented above.[10]

These comparative drawings are followed by a list of 97 'diseases' which medical authorities, whose names are attached to each entry, ascribed to the wearing of stays and corsets. They are divided into complaints of the head, the chest, the abdomen, and 'general', and include sleepiness, apoplexy, whooping-cough, consumption, ugly children, dropsy of the belly, and epilepsy.[11]

'Luke Limner Esq' had evidently read widely. He had discovered Daniel Chodoweiki's 'natural forms' of dress which had been published in the *Frauenzimmer Almanach* of 1785,[12] as well as strictures on the vagaries of the fashions of their times by writers of classical Rome ranging from Plautus to Tertullian. He had found too sumptuary laws issued at various later periods of history, including those of Pope Urban viii in 1635.[13] He claimed that 'The Gout even, is said to have aided *le gout*; the broad-toed and slashed shoes of Henry viii being attributed to a royal malady'.[14]

Most of the trouble he ascribed to the inadequate education offered to women and their consequent

deficiency of mental acquirements. .... As a class-book, for the heads of families and governesses in particular, we would recommend – *The Principles of Physiology, applied to the preservation of Health*, by Andrew Combe M.D., a work that if read with care could not fail to contribute a powerful influence in modifying the received opinions of the innoxious effects of the corset and of its indispensable improvement of the female natural form.[15]

This is the book, published in 1834, which had run into fourteen editions by 1852. The recommendation of it more than twenty years later shows that its principles still seemed relevant.

Although desperately anxious to persuade women to abandon the dangerous corset, 'Luke Limner' was evidently no feminist, for he recognised that it might, indeed, have its negative uses:

it would prevent Females with stronger heads, than understanding, walking our hospitals – as tight corsets might prevent 'Sweet Girl Graduates' from solving problems in the Occult sciences.[16]

Madre Natura had no difficulty in discerning the evil in current fashions and, as well, in those recently gone out; high heels, crinolettes (today called 'bustles'), chignons, and tight-lacing were all both dangerous to health and ugly; but she pointed to no alternative outline that might have been followed for a more desirable form of dress. Praxiteles would have rejected the crinolette; but what would he have liked 19th-century English women to wear? We are not told. Luke Limner could draw Madre Natura's perfect feminine skeleton, but he could not clothe it. In 1874 a stereotype for aesthetic and hygienic dress had not yet been circulated though it had been designed.

By this time indeed, clothes by which artistic, strong-minded, or platform women could be recognised were beginning to appear. There must always have been some women in any society who had preferred clothes which were original in design. Mrs Nassau Senior, for instance, in her portrait by Watts painted in 1858,[17] wears a very uncommon dress which conveys no more than that she was a woman of taste; [9] but the clothes of the progressively minded little Mrs Duncombe in Charlotte Yonge's novel *Three Brides*, published in 1876, are certainly meant to belong to a recognisable *type* of woman, though they bear no label. Mrs Duncombe was small and slim when, in 1876, it was fashionable for women to be Phidian in appearance. She was also daring in her behaviour for, although she was fairly acceptable in good society, she had risen to her feet at a village meeting arranged to discuss its sanitation, and had expressed an opinion and one, moreover, which differed from that of the Chairman – the local M.P. and landowner.

It is clear that not only those at the meeting but also the author herself thought that this behaviour was extraordinary. Mrs Duncombe ought to have got her husband to voice her views for her but he was a racing-man and opposed to views. Her character established, Mrs Duncombe's clothes are described. Cecilia, one of the ladies present at the meeting was surprised at Mrs Duncombe's mode of dress:

> She would have taken Miss Slater for the strong-minded woman rather than this small slim person, with the complexion going with the yellower species of red hair and chignon not unlike a gold-pheasant's, while the thin aquiline nose made Cecilia think of Queen Elizabeth. The dress was tight-fitting black silk, with a gorgeous many-coloured, gold-embroidered oriental mantle thrown loosely over it, a Tyrolean hat, about as large as the pheasant's comb, tipped over her forehead, with cords and tassels of gold; she made little restless movements . . . And before the astonished eyes of the meeting, the gold-pheasant hopped upon the platform, and with as much ease as if she had been Queen Bess dragooning her parliament, she gave what even the astounded gentlemen felt to be a sensible, practical exposition of ways and means.[18]

Mrs Duncombe was not the heroine of *Three Brides*, that would have been impossible. She was a little ridiculous but the author treats her with compassion. When she invited the gentry to dinner in the modest villa which was all her gambling husband, a retired Captain, could manage, it is made plain that she was no housekeeper and that her two boys were badly brought-up. Nevertheless, although the menu went wrong and the sons were rude, the dinner was a success. While the company waited for their host and hostess to appear, two of the guests withdrew into a 'small conservatory or glazed niche . . . The place contained two desolate camellias . . . and one scraggy leafless geranium . . . the Venus de Milo stood on a bracket, with a riding-whip in her arms, and a bundle of working-society tickets behind her, and her *vis à vis* the Faun of Praxiteles was capped with a glove with one finger pointing upwards'.[19] Mrs Duncombe and her husband at last appeared, 'the lady as usual picturesque, though in the old black silk, with a Roman sash tied transversely, and holly in her hair'.[20] All this is surely Charlotte Yonge at her very best.

The dinner had been given to introduce an American clergyman and his wife, an advocate of women's rights who was invited to lead an after-dinner discussion on the 'Equality of the Sexes':

> 'Women purify the atmosphere wherever they go', said the lady.
> 'Many women do', returned Julius, 'but will they retain that power universally if they succeed in obtaining the position where there will be less consideration for them, and they must be exposed to a certain hardening and roughening process?'[21]

We are back in the *Woman's World* of eight years earlier.

Apart from its conventionally romantic aspects the two themes of the *Three Brides* – women's rights and healthy drains – were both fashionable: the drains led to an outbreak of typhus in the village in which not only villagers but some of the gentry who nursed them died; the rights of women were confined to the sort of discussion quoted above. Mrs Duncombe proved to have been wrong-headed in her views on sanitation and suffered a further downfall with the bankruptcy of her husband. She fades out of the book before the end, via conversion to the Church of Rome.

In 1876 Charlotte Yonge had contented herself with labelling Mrs Duncombe's appearance 'picturesque'. In 1870 Benjamin Disraeli had published his heady *Lothair* and swept up his reader into higher circles than Miss Yonge had ever ventured to explore. They were inhabited by Cardinals, Dukes and, we must believe, from the coolness with which he viewed them – by the author himself. No character of Disraeli's could have been so coarse as to appear 'picturesque', nor could the author have been so imprecise in describing a member of his cast, all of whom either fed upon ortolans in aspic or rejected them as too banal and called for cold meat. Even the elderly women were very beautiful and the young ones proportionally more so. Of the three heroines, all of them perfect, one, Mrs Campian far surpassed the others.

Theodora Campian was thought of as being Roman by race; when Lothair first caught sight of her at a dinner party she was wearing her habitual expression

if not of disdain, of extreme reserve ... pale but perfectly Attic in outline, with the short upper-lip, and the round chin, and a profusion of dark chestnut hair bound by a Grecian fillet, and on her brow a star.[22]

Although still young, when she appears in the novel Theodora is mature. However, we are told that at seventeen she had served as model for the head of Liberty on the five-franc piece of a short-lived French Republic. This establishes both her type and the world she moved in. Lothair

thought he had never seen anyone or anything so serene ... what one pictures of Olympian repose. And the countenance was Olympian: a Phidian face with large grey eyes and dark lashes; wonderful hair abounding without art and gathered into Grecian fillets.[23]

Mrs Campian and her American husband moved correctly in English society. Their own circle included a successful painter, Mr Phoebus: "'I fancied", said Lothair to Mr Phoebus, watching Mrs Campian glide out of the pavilion ... "I had heard that Mrs Campian was a Roman."'

'The Romans were Greeks', said Mr Phoebus, 'and in this instance the Phidian type came out.'
'I fear the Phidian type is very rare,' said Lothair.
'In nature and in art there must always be surpassing instances', said Mr Phoebus.[24]

Commissioned by the Czar of Russia, Mr Phoebus painted a *Hero and Leander*, which he was graciously permitted to exhibit in London before despatching it to St Petersburg. It revealed

a figure of life-size, exhibiting in undisguised completeness the ... female form and yet the painter had so skilfully availed himself of the shadowy and mystic hour and some gauze-like drapery, which veiled without concealing his design that the chastest eye might gaze on his heroine with impunity.[25]

It is not overtly stated that Theodora Campian had sat for *Hero*, that would have suggested immodesty, but the 'Phidian type' appeared in its purest nineteenth-century form in Disraeli's descriptions both of Theodora Campian and of Mr Phoebus's *Hero*. The type had already been painted by Lord Leighton in his *Greek Girl dancing* of 1867 and it was to appear on many canvases both by him and by his contemporaries before he fatally caricatured it in his *Last Watch of Hero* of 1889. Only a little later, at the beginning of the 1890s, George du Maurier modified the type very slightly for his French laundry girl, Trilby; and by this time Mrs Langtry, the 'Jersey Lily' with the 'short upper-lip and the round chin', had become the most-talked of beauty in England. Greek beauty had a long innings, certainly due in part to its appearance of vigorous health in an age that was greatly concerned with the dangers of sickness in over-crowded conditions.

As for Mrs Campian's 'Grecian fillets', they were the one feature of the new taste in dress that could be identified as early as the end of the 'sixties. Before the publication of *Lothair* they had already appeared in *Punch*; and in 1869 Thomas Armstrong exhibited in the Royal Academy a painting of three young women, manifestly portraits, standing in a hayfield. [Frontispiece] All three wear dresses of extremely simple cut and their hair, gathered into a knot at the nape of the neck, is bound with fillets in the Grecian style. The dresses of the young women in Armstrong's *Hay Time* (who wear aprons and hold rakes but are certainly not peasants) appear to be unrelated to the current fashion, but they are not. The picture must have been painted in that brief interval between the disappearance of the crinoline and the arrival of the Watteau toilette, when fashionable women wore straight dresses with a long train as do the haymakers – that is to say, in the summer of 1868. However fashionable the composition of the dresses, the stuff of which they are made could not have been bought in a shop of the period; although basically linen or perhaps cotton, one dress is embroidered all over in a pattern of flowers and leaves, the other is probably hand-printed from a woodblock.

The unconventional appearance of these girls (rather pretty to our eyes) may have provoked the disapproval expressed about the painting. Discussing it in his notice of the Royal Academy exhibition which was published on May 12th, the art critic of the *Owl* wrote:

Hay Time. Three very plain persons who, having evidently not made hay while the sun shone, are now doing it by moonlight.[26]

The art critic of the *Owl* either did not, or pretended he did not, recognise the 'plain persons' for what they actually were – exponents of ultimate refinement in tasteful dress. It would be difficult to account for the meandering pattern on the stuff worn by the girl on the spectator's left except as a very early example of the crewel-work that was to become a craze in artistic circles during the 1870s. This embroidery in loosely twisted wools of muted colours, resembling the products of natural dyes, was usually worked on thin wool or linen or cotton sheeting (often unbleached), and had ousted the stiff mid-Victorian patterns of brilliantly coloured full-blown roses, closely bunched together, that had been embroidered in 'Berlin work' as chair-seats and fire-screens and were by the end of the 'sixties considered vulgar.

In 1877, nearly ten years after the date of the clothes worn in *Hay Time*, the *Queen*, not a magazine of advanced ideas, presented its readers with a supplement in the form of a coloured print of trailing convolvulus sprays, intended as a design for a crewel-work decoration on a tennis-apron. The flowers, sparsely and gracefully springing from fine wandering stems are, in style and spacing, very much like the pattern worn by the *Hay Time* girl. It was the first of a succession of such designs published or advocated by the *Queen* during the last three years of the 'seventies.

Later in 1877, the year of the tennis-apron embroidery, the *Queen* reviewed favourably a new novel by Mrs Oliphant, *Carita*, the theme of which is expounded by three generations of middle-class women, one old, one in middle-life and one a girl. At one point in the story Miss Cherry, a middle-aged virgin, and her youthful niece, Cara, persuade a young neighbour, Edward, to read to them from the *Idylls of the King* – *Elaine* to be precise – while they occupy their hands with needlework. Miss Cherry explains

> It is a new kind of needlework, Edward. I dont know if you have seen any of it. It is considered a great deal better in design than the Berlin work we used to do, and it is a very easy stitch and goes quickly. That is what I like in it . . . but I am not sure that I dont prefer the Berlin work. After all, to work borders to dusters seems scarcely worth while, does it? O yes, my dear, I know it is for a chair; but it looks just like a duster. Now we used to work on silk and satin – much better worth it.[27]

So Mrs Oliphant places her Miss Cherry, up from the country and ignorant of the sensibilities of the new middle-class intellectuals whose taste was for simplicity rather than opulence, as even the *Queen* had begun to perceive.

It is clear that by 1877, as a means of describing a recognisable group of ideas that amounted to the current taste, the word 'art' had become serviceable, though it had not yet, apparently, been applied to the dress worn by people to whom Art was important. Charlotte Yonge was using the word 'picturesque' for the clothes of Mrs Duncombe, with her casts of the Venus de Milo and the Praxiteles Faun in her neglected conservatory; Disraeli had not labelled the dress of Theodora Campian, although he twice referred to her 'Grecian fillets' which were not worn with the hairdressing dictated by Paris in 1870 when *Lothair* was written. However, in 1878 the *Queen*, which had a large circulation, evidently considered the new taste in dress sufficiently important to be worth discussing at length. Having reviewed, the previous year, a book with the title of *The Art of Beauty* by Mrs Haweis, the editor must have decided that she was the right person to discuss the particular kind of dress that was seen to be increasingly worn by women of a minority group in the society of the time – a dress that had a homogeneity of design. So the *Queen* published three articles by her with the general title of *PreRaphaelite Dress*. It is hardly necessary to point out that by this time the PreRaphaelite movement itself was far from new; indeed, although its influence remained, it was technically dead.

Mrs Haweis was the wife of a clergyman whose sermons were fashionable but whose income was not large enough to provide the background that his wife needed in order to express her personal taste in dress and furnishings. Her taste in dress seems to have been both expensive and what she herself described as eccentric. In picking Mrs Haweis to write about new ideas in dress the *Queen* chose well; she was admirably equipped to explain to those just outside the central ring what was going on inside it. She had a pretty little talent for drawing and, as well as designing covers for her husband's religious publications in the advanced style in decorative art of the day, she had illustrated works by other authors. Neither a prophet nor an innovator she understood perfectly what was going on, and had she lived today would probably have been a very well-paid fashion-journalist on a high-class Sunday paper. It is possible that she knew enough to jib a little at using the term PreRaphaelite at all as late as 1878 – the choice was probably the *Queen's* – but once she had adopted it she continued to use it.

'I am sometimes asked', began Mrs Haweis,

what is meant by 'PreRaphaelitism in Dress' . . . we may say in a general way that the present movement in dress under the above name, which is gradually spreading, first among art circles who have discovered, then among aesthetic circles who appreciate, the laws which govern beauty, represents the common reaction which follows any bad system carried on too long. Fashions generally begin well, fall into hideous extravagance, then a reaction to this extravagance and so on *ad infinitum*.[28]

There follow examples from the past, for Mrs Haweis, like her distinguished contemporary, James Planché, the retired Somerset Herald, was a historian of dress. Planché's famous *Cyclopaedia of Costume* appeared in 1880.[29] Mrs Haweis continued:

The primary rule in a beautiful dress is that it shall not contradict the natural form of the human frame ... One of the most important features in a graceful figure – hence one of the most conspicuous and valuable innovations of the PreRaphaelite School – is the waist. The first aim is to have an 'antique waist' – which a vulgar mind would pronounce horribly thick – thick like the Venus de Medicis, thick like that of the far nobler Venus de Milo ... The waist of the PreRaphaelite is rather short – where a waist ought to be in fact, between the hips and the last rib ... Her sleeves are cut extraordinarily high on the shoulder, sometimes a little fulled to fit the shoulder bone; for it is *de rigeur* that a PreRaphaelite should be capable of moving her arms as freely when dressed as when undressed. As to walking dresses, the PreRaphaelite is very wise, and very independent of vulgar opinion. She selects good sensible forms and keeps to them ... the PreRaphaelite defies fashion whenever it is bad; but she goes along with it if it mends its ways and becomes good.[30] [Headpiece to Chapter 5]

In her second article Mrs Haweis discussed colour:

The so-called 'PreRaphaelites' whom I have before shown to be not worshippers of one period, but the humble seekers after the laws of beauty in art, have so far influenced intelligent public opinion, and hence trade, that an immense number of really beautiful colours have become purchasable, and even fashionable, of late years. 'No colour harmony', said Ruskin many years ago, 'is of a high order unless it involve indescribable tints' ...[31]

Mrs Haweis goes on to list colours which are not indescribable and which are, therefore bad. White is an example she gives.

It is doubtful whether Mrs Haweis herself often wore
PreRaphaelite dress. It was not quite her *genre*, as she might
have put it. Descriptions of the gowns she did wear appear
frequently in her letters, and they sound a good deal grander
than the kind of artistic dress embellished with crewel-work
that aimed at simplicity. Of the size of her waist she says
nothing, but the creations she wore at the royal Drawing-rooms
she often attended do not sound as though they would have
suited the Venus de Milo. They were usually of rich silk
brocade, often in ivory colour, their long trains edged with
brown velvet and decorated with ruchings or festoons of hand-
made Brussels lace. True, they seem to have followed the
straight line, called 'princess' at the end of the 1870s, but this
was, at the time, the latest composition produced by the Paris
haute couture. If her wardrobe included 'indescribable tints'
she does not seem to have had much difficulty in finding
general names for them.

When Mrs Haweis decided to be 'eccentric' in her dress it
was perhaps natural that, as a historian of the clothing of the
past, she should have chosen to imitate some earlier fashions.
She speaks, for instance, of a dress she designed for one of her
own musical evenings, made in the style of a Court lady of
Charles II's time and in Japanese brocade lined with orange.
On this combination of orient and occident she does not
comment. In 1876 she wrote to her mother of the effect that
she and her little son were making during a visit to Mr and
Mrs Cowper Temple:

> The ladies dress beautifully ... my eccentric dresses make
> me quite celebrated I find, and Lionel keeps up the reputa-
> tion of the family.

Lionel, who was at that time five or six years old,

> is much improved and creates a great sensation by his beauty
> and genius. He has an early Charles II dress and an Early
> English one. The first is made of crimson velvet slashed with
> white and trimmed with antique lace and sable and the other
> white blanketing trimmed with gold embroidery.[32]

The Art of Dress, her second book, which Mrs Haweis completed in 1879, included some material from her articles in the *Queen*. She also reproduced some of 'Luke Limner's' diagrams (Luke Limner was in fact John Leighton) and she devoted a few paragraphs to fashions of the past, reproducing an engraving of a fifteenth century horned head-dress also used by Planché. Like most writers of her generation she was prepared to state her views as facts and to deduce from them a code of morality to be applied to dress – an attitude of mind inseparable, it seems, from the growing optimism of the last quarter of the 19th century.

A simple garb usually springs from simple manners while a complex social state and a lowered *morale* fly to furbelows and 'intemperance in ornament' but we must distinguish between real and affected simplicity, such as the unrobed Lely beauties and the misrobed 'shepherdesses' that appeared in George II's time.[33]

Mrs Haweis saw danger in fashions in decay, she feared the dying fall, and saw that what had been charming could turn sour. While she agreed with Mrs Bloomer that the hooped underskirt was a comfort in windy weather, 'as we all found when it first appeared about 1850; but too large a one is an undeniable nuisance'.[34] From this she drew a philosophy and concluded that 'Coarse vulgar curves, unmeaning lumps, superabundant ornament ... are to be avoided' –[35] as were many other fashions of dress, especially those found in fashions in decay or, in less emotional language, the style that was at the moment on the way out.

For in 1879 lumps, as exemplified by the gathered-up folds of the Watteau toilette, held out over a crinolette, were already out of fashion and replaced, temporarily, as the crinoline had been ten years earlier, by a mermaid-like composition which clung to the body and spread into a fan-like tail that lay on the ground behind. This fashion lasted about three years, longer than the two or three months enjoyed by its predecessor in the late 'sixties. It was itself replaced in the 1880s by more lumps.

'If,' wrote Mrs Haweis, 'we are wearing, as at present, a costume which (when not overdone) is really good, it is but fair to say so';[36] and she was able to justify her partiality for the 'princess' line by showing, in a diagram, that it followed the natural lines of the female body. [16] Seen from the front and when the wearer stood upright with her feet together this was undeniably true, especially if, by slightly bending one knee and thereby shifting the weight from a strictly vertical position, a gentle but by no means vulgar curve could be achieved. The fashion, however, had its disadvantages, for to be seen at its best the skirt had to be fastened behind the knees by hidden interior ties which induced it to cling to the legs in front. Together with a line of demarcation round the hips, this imparted a pleasing hint of the draperies of the Venus of Milos while permitting the actual waist to be held discreetly in to a circumference elegantly smaller than Venus's; but the dress was neither comfortable nor easy to wear for those who lacked the poise to manage it. [17, 19] Mrs Haweis rather unfairly revealed the fact that a really expensive dressmaker could cut the dress so skilfully that no interior ties were necessary, but she did not disguise the truth that such a cut was not within the reach of everybody.[37]

In her *Art of Dress* of 1879 Mrs Haweis included a drawing of hair held by what in the late 1860s would have been named 'Grecian fillets', which is, she says, 'one of the prettiest methods of doing up the hair . . . affected greatly by the artistic world'.[38] Rather surprisingly she says that this is, 'a revival of the mediaeval fashion, properly Prae-Raphaelite . . . The classic arrangement of the hair, such as we see in statues of both male and female deities . . . is also simulated by Prae-Raphaelite ladies nowadays'.[39]

The spelling 'Prae-Raphaelite' she adopted specially for this book.

Although the word 'gothic' was, apparently, never to be heard in the sartorial language of the 1870s, the adjective PreRaphaelite was probably often used by young couples shopping for their future homes, and married women must have resorted to it in trying to explain their ideas to inexpensive dressmakers. It was certainly not the pallid flat-cheeked girls with startling curved lips immortalised by Rossetti and Swinburne who moved the arbiters of taste of the 'seventies, but the great torso and compact head of the Venus of Milos though she was, indeed, rather too late for the moment they thought of as perfect.

Now the culminating age in the life of ancient Greece I call beyond question, a great epoch; the life of Athens in the fifth century before our era I call one of the highly developed, one of the marking, one of the modern periods in the life of the whole human race . . . The Athenians, Thucydides says, had given up, although not very long before, an extravagance of dress and an excess of personal ornament which, in the first flush of a newly-discovered luxury, had been adopted by some of the richer classes.

It was Matthew Arnold who drew, in 1869, this parallel between Athens and the enlightened section of English Victorian society.[40] William Frederick Farrar, Dean of Canterbury, however, disliked what he saw, and wrote in 1875: 'a corrupt Hellenism which regards sin forsooth with aesthetic toleration . . .'[41]

Even practical Mrs Haweis saw that in Victorian England Greek dress would never do, although she admitted that it was

the most perfect of known costume . . . The Greek pallium, sufficiently padded to brave an English climate would be too heavy to be popular and far too expensive for the poorer classes . . . the Greek chyton might be made to display and to protect . . . but it would limit us to clinging fabrics, which would ensure revolt from those who properly see charm in glossy, slippery and even massive velvet materials, all of which are unfit for *toga* or *tunica*; and it would tend to depress trade by thus cutting off various branches of industry.[42]

How true. Yet how different from the high-toned discussions in the *Woman's World* at the end of the Serious 'Sixties when aesthetics and dress were rarely mentioned.

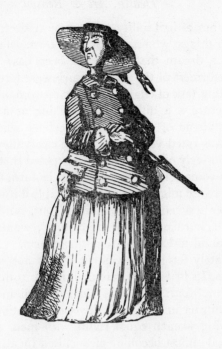

4

The Strong-minded Woman

Efforts towards a reform in the design of women's dress were
entangled so inextricably in the 19th century with organised
struggles for the rights of women that the first cannot be
properly understood without some understanding of the second.

Intellectual supporters of the rights of women could see that
while their opponents regarded women as too frail, both
physically and mentally (and perhaps even morally), to endure
any added responsibilities, it was never suggested that they
should grow more robust. On the contrary, most middle-class
Englishmen dreamed of women who, far from being robust,
were tender and gentle; whose soft voices could smooth away

their patches of irritability and whose desires, if women must have such things, would mirror their own.

It was a dream that has never been easy to disperse, but women reformers of the 19th century were forced to tackle the unrewarding task of edging this dream-woman from the centre of the picture – a difficult undertaking at a time when the Christian virtue of selflessness, especially when practised by women, was rated very high. Every effort they made to enter fields exclusively occupied by men exposed them to the accusation of unwomanliness – which led, in its turn, to the suggestion that their cause might be more acceptable if it were represented by prettier women. It was pointed out, however, that since public life 'hardened the countenance', women who entered it were bound to lose their feminine charm.

Fortunately for the movement it was not solely dependent on women. Its first crucial moment in the 19th century arrived when John Stuart Mill was elected Parliamentary Member for Westminster in 1865 with the open intention of introducing a Bill giving women equal rights with men. As it happened, women had almost become enfranchised by an oversight which would have allowed them to benefit from the reading of 'man' as 'mankind' in the 1867 Second Reform Bill. This was discovered in time to prevent so dramatic a happening on a large scale though a few small groups of women did manage to vote at the polls here and there. The wording was soon clarified, and later in 1867 Mill proposed in the House of Commons the granting of the Suffrage to such women as were single, or widowed and householders in their own right, as an amendment to the Representation of the People Act of 1867. His amendment was defeated but it had the support of eighty-one Members of the House, including both Conservatives and Liberals. Enthusiasts for the cause were, naturally, much encouraged, and *Woman's World* must certainly have come into being as a result of the number of declared sympathisers who, together with those outside Parliament, should have been sufficient to keep such a weekly going. Three years later, in 1870, the *Woman's Suffrage Journal* was launched under the editorship of Miss Lydia Becker who was long to be a supporter of the women's movement, and who had, as will be seen later, decided views on the way women should dress.

This is not the place to review in detail the particular phase of the Women's Rights movement that began with Mill's election to Parliament in 1865 and long survived his defeat in the following election of 1868, but the names of at least some of the women associated with it are important. The Garrett sisters, Elizabeth, Millicent and Agnes, the first two to become Elizabeth Garrett Anderson and Millicent Fawcett, were among them, and so was a cousin, Rhoda Garrett, an artist. There was Barbara Leigh Smith who, first unmarried and later as Madame Bodichon, was admired by Rossetti who met her in the house of mutual friends; Emily Davies, to be associated with her in the founding of Girton College; John Bright's two sisters, three daughters and three nieces; Thackeray's daughter, later Lady Ritchie; Josephine Butler, Florence Nightingale, and Elizabeth Barrett Browning. If these are among the names best remembered today, many women equally distinguished and innumerable others less so, supported the movement from the beginning of the John Stuart Mill epoch, for he must be regarded as, in the words of Millicent Fawcett,

a master who formed a school of thought, just as in art, a master forms a school and influences his successors for generations ... One great service of Mill to the women's movement in England has been, I conceive, in impressing upon it from the first, the character of practical good sense and moderation that has been its distinguishing feature.[1]

Portraits, drawings, engravings, and even photographs of many of the women who were most active in the late 1860s have survived. From their looks and their dress it seems that Mill's 'good sense and moderation' guided their taste. It is difficult to find any outward trace of the masculine woman dreaded (or hoped for as a target) by opponents of their enfranchisement. In the National Portrait Gallery is a touching painting by Ford Madox Brown of Henry Fawcett and his wife Millicent. Her golden-red hair, of the colour so much admired by the PreRaphaelites, is dressed in the fashion of the moment – the painting must have been done in 1867 – and she sits perched on the arm of her husband's chair, her arm round his shoulders, her dark grey dress livened by a splash of colour as it is caught up, apparently by accident, so that her red crinolined underskirt shows.

Henry Fawcett, in spite of an accident at the age of twenty-five which resulted in complete and permanent blindness, was elected Member of Parliament for Brighton in 1865. He presided in 1868 (a year after his marriage) at one of the series of weekly meetings on the subject of female suffrage held in a church hall in Blackfriars Road. It was what *The Times* described, the next day, as his 'lengthy and elaborate address' that occasioned not only a long report of the meeting at which, according to the reporter, 'the audience was very numerous and, as might be expected, comprised a large contingent of fair aspirants to electoral franchise',[2] but also a leader in the same issue, April 9th.

By this time the 'strong-minded woman' had long been an image in the mind of the public. Miss Deborah Jenkins was described by Mrs Gaskell in her novel *Cranford*, published in 1850, as having a 'strong mind'. Miss Deborah, though on the side of the angels, was presented by the author as a distinctly obstinate woman. In 1859 Jane Carlyle declared in a letter, that she noticed 'a growing taste for fastness or, worse still, strong-mindedness' in women.[3] Miss Braddon's 'I dont want a strong-minded woman who writes books and wears green spectacles',[4] spread the concept through her popular novel, *Lady Audley's Secret* of 1862.

Later, in her *Three Brides*, published in 1876, Charlotte Yonge's conventional Cecilia expressed surprise, as we have seen, that her 'platform woman' did not look typically strong-minded, which makes it clear that she had a definite picture of a strong-minded woman in her head; she had, in fact, picked out a Miss Slater for the role – Miss Slater had worn black. In this instance one suspects that the clothes actually chosen by Miss Yonge for her progressive Mrs Duncombe were partly

based on those worn by Madame Bodichon who was photographed in the late 'sixties wearing a burnous-like mantle
which she had brought back from Algeria, though Madame
Bodichon was wealthy and Mrs Duncombe the reverse.

It had been about Madame Bodichon, before her marriage,
that Rossetti had written to his sister:

> Ah if you were only like Miss Barbara Leigh Smith, a young
> lady I meet at the Howetts blessed with large rations of tin,
> fat, enthusiasm and golden hair who thinks nothing of
> climbing a mountain in breeches or wading through a
> stream in none in the name of sacred pigment.[5]

Miss Leigh Smith painted. Both in her photograph in the
burnous and in a drawing of her head Madame Bodichon looks
pretty in a piquant way but in neither does she look fat unless,
perhaps, in contrast to the gaunt Christina Rossetti. Her 'tin'
Madame Bodichon used to endow Girton College. She may
indeed have worn breeches to climb mountains but in the lively
little drawings that show her on the wind-swept heights she
wears a jacket and skirt with a big hat, exactly like the country
clothes that Effie Ruskin had worn in the Highlands a decade
or so earlier. [22] It is hard to believe that this was the kind of
girl to be dreaded as a corrupting influence.

If the Opposition's vision of the strong-minded woman is
difficult to discover as a historic personage, the disapproving
newspaper reports are consistent in their description of her
appearance, and these are confirmed by illustrations to jokes
at her expense in *Punch*. In these her hair is usually cut short to
the nape of her neck (it varies a little in its actual length) and
her dress is dark, severe and often includes the kind of square-
cut jacket that was obviously appropriate to the country gentry
but wrong in town. [Headpiece to Chapter 4]

It is natural that women with lively and fully occupied
minds should have found it irksome to conform rigidly to the
fashions in dress worn by the majority of conventional women.
Even the constant changes of fashion itself seemed to symbolise
infirmity of purpose to those whose ambition it was to appear
sufficiently stable and reliable to be entrusted with the Vote,

but since fashion is invincible, those who tried to escape it in their dress found themselves and their ideas caught up and swept along as a part of its stream. Even the image of the strong-minded woman devised by newspaper reporters, Opposition Members of Parliament, and artists employed by *Punch*, could not resist the torrent. [23] Unless they presented her in clothes that had gone out of fashion, in which case she became a harmless back-number and therefore indistinguishable among the hordes of ordinary women similarly dressed, they could only envisage her wearing a costume entirely composed of those elements of the current fashion that reflected masculine dress. The trouble was that since the fashion had abandoned the sweetness of the crinoline period and grown more bold, certain masculine elements could be found in the dress even of those dove-like creatures who were most approved of by the conventional male. The young Ellen Terry – and at no moment in her life could she be accused of strong-mindedness – wore her hair cut short; the Princess of Wales, so much admired for her gentle beauty, wore on occasion a boater and a masculine collar and tie; many of the most elegant women wore black. [21]

If, taken singly, these masculine features could add a pleasing accent to a toilette otherwise wholly feminine, assembled as the dress of a hollow-cheeked, ageing woman in pince-nez they could serve as a warning to sweet things to keep away from politics – particularly when the *Saturday Review* assured them that 'they know – and it is surprising that Mr Fawcett does not know it too – that a woman could not touch that [political] pitch without being defiled'.[6]

In 1868 the *Saturday Review*, while determined to be fashionably censorious of empty-headed, idle women, produced, in a long article on Feminine Affectations, the most vivid verbal description that has survived of the strong-minded woman. It was not, apparently, only the clothes she wore but her behaviour, too, that marked her mannishness. In contrast to the idle vapid woman is, says the *Saturday Review*

the mannish woman who wears a double breasted coat with

big buttons, of which she flings back the lapels with an air, understanding the suggestiveness of a wide chest and the need of unchecked breathing; who wears unmistakeable shirt fronts, linen collars, vests and plain ties, like a man; who folds her arms or sets them akimbo, like a man; who even nurses her feet and cradles her knees, in spite of her petticoats, and makes believe that the attitude is comfortable because it is manlike. If the excessively womanly woman is affected in her sickly sweetness, the mannish woman is affected in her breadth and roughness ... She rounds her elbows and turns her wrist outward, as men round their elbows and turn their wrists outward ... and in contrast with the intensely womanly woman, who uses the tips of her fingers only, the mannish woman when she does anything uses her whole hand, and if she had to thread a needle would thread it as much by her palm as by her fingers. All of which is affectation, from first to last affectation; a mere assumption of virile fashions utterly inharmonious to the whole being, physical and mental, of a woman.[7]

This female, the *Saturday Review* also pointed out, loved dogs above children, was a good shot, lingered over beer and cheese, and tossed off wine instead of timidly sipping it. It can hardly have been an accident that the *Saturday Review's* analysis of feminine affectations coincided with the presentation of the Bill for the Married Women's Property Act in June 1868: its stereotype of the strong-minded woman was not readily forgotten. During the Parliamentary debate on the Bill, those who opposed it had stressed the fact that while some women deserved to be treated as rational beings, there were those who did not. Already in the same year the *Times* had suggested that 'the ambiguous phalanx will be an object of disgust to both sexes';[8] and the portrait of the supposed member of the phalanx was eventually to be filled out in the House itself, especially by Mr Smollett, a descendant of the novelist, who opposed the enfranchisement of women. Mr Smollett had been rebuked by *Punch* in April 1868 for being very severe on everybody and using 'language which does not seem out of place in Roderick

Random but which the author's descendant might have made a little more decorous for the House of Commons'.[9] He was, before long, to use stronger language still.

In the meantime both the *Times* and *Punch* had agreed that the conduct of the ladies in the gallery during the debate on the Married Women's Property Bill had not been impeccable. *Punch* reported that 'the Ladies in the "Cage" above the reporters made all sorts of disturbances during the debate, such as murmuring, hissing, clapping hands and rattling fans against the brass. Mr Punch thinks, with all submission, that they had better confine such demonstrations to the theatre.'[10]

The Married Women's Property Bill got through its first reading: the Petition for the Enfranchisement of Women, signed by 21,757 women headed by Mrs Somerville and Florence Nightingale and presented to the House by John Stuart Mill, had no effect. There, so far as the House was concerned, the matter rested until 1875 when the second reading of the Women's Disabilities Removal Bill was presented by Mr Forsyth in April. Mr Smollett's speech in opposition to this Bill was described as including language too coarse to be repeated. It was, of course, reported in *Hansard*, though whether with modifications is difficult to determine. Mr Smollett, it appears, claimed that

the agitation was brought into Great Britain by an importation of turbulent women from America where it had been going on without any good result for something like half a century. Those ladies came over to champion 'Woman's Rights', and proclaim the equality of the sexes; and to show they had a right to do so they assumed, or rather usurped, male attire – they clad themselves in breeches. They were called 'Bloomers' . . . women made use of this dress as an attraction to the male sex, for there is nothing so pleasing to the latter as a well-dressed woman. The ladies soon discovered that the new costume was not attractive. They saw at once that the pectoral, abdominal, and fundamental development of the sex looked grotesque in male attire. That style of dress was therefore soon abandoned. But although this distinctive dress was discontinued, the type of the strong-minded woman still survived.[11]

The link between 'mannish' and 'strong-minded' was thus strengthened. Mr Smollett was supported by Mr Leatham who added:

The House may at once gather the real scope and object of this movement if it recalls what took place last year.

For when the exclusion of married women from the franchise had been discussed,

There was an immediate exclamation, I will not call it a 'shriek' from the sisterhood . . .[12]

In the highly charged atmosphere that surrounded debates on women's suffrage nothing escaped unnoticed. Mr Leatham's speech may soon have been forgotten but the epithet 'shrieking sisterhood' passed into the language. It was used in 1890 in a bad-tempered and muddled book by James McGrigor Allan titled *Women's Suffrage Wrong*, and it was used with pride by women themselves during the Women's Suffrage struggles in the first decade of the 20th century.

In 1874 the *Graphic* included a steel-engraving of the occupants of the platform at a meeting in the Hanover Rooms, arranged in preparation for the presentation of the Women's Disabilities Removal Bill that would so inflame Mr Smollett the following year. [25] In the engraving ladies in the front row are identified by their names, inscribed beneath each of them – the gentlemen are not. On the left is Millicent Fawcett; behind the table in the centre is Lydia Becker, who had been mentioned in *Woman's World* as reading a paper to the British Association in 1868 and had become first editor of the *Women's Suffrage Journal* soon afterwards; on her feet, facing the spectators and addressing the meeting, is Miss Rhoda Garrett who wears her hair long to her shoulders and held back from her face by the kind of band worn by Lewis Carroll's 'Alice'. Miss Garrett is plainly dressed in a double-breasted square-cut jacket with big buttons, a kerchief is knotted round her neck. She is, moreover, distinctly pretty. To what category was she thought of as belonging? Her jacket undoubtedly conforms to the *Saturday Review's* account of that worn by the mannish woman, and also to Effie Ruskin's and Madame Bodichon's country-wear of years before. Miss Garrett was an artist; was she 'being', if anything, just that? Or had the *Graphic's* illustrator imposed on her the regulation uniform of the platform woman?

The *Saturday Review* had unwittingly provided at least one clue to the survival of the strong-minded woman in describing her gesture of flinging back her double-breasted jacket with its big buttons as 'understanding the suggestiveness of a wide chest and the need of unchecked breathing'. In this need the phalanx had the opinion of the whole of the medical profession behind it. Doctors, 'Luke Limner Esq.' and Mrs Haweis, had all of them spared no pains in demonstrating in words, and diagrams the urgent necessity of reforming the dress of women so that their ribs could have freedom to expand and their lungs to fill with air. Strong-minded women, it seems, even if only as fictional characters, responded.

Fit enough, however, for physical survival, the strong-minded women of the 1870s were still to face several decades of hostile criticism. In 1884, for instance, the *Nineteenth Century*, a forward-looking periodical which was sensitive and adventurous in its choice of contributors and topics, published an article on the Platform Woman by Margaret Lonsdale. In spite of the fact that during the same year the *Nineteenth Century* was printing a considerable number of serious articles by women – among them Octavia Hill on Colour, Space and Music for the People, and Rosalind Marryat on the pollution of water by sewer-gas – Miss Lonsdale was against the platform woman:

The mental and moral condition which the modern platform woman herself exhibits, is the surest proof of the mischief which public speaking is working by her agency in the community at large – the gradual hardening of the countenance and of the external manner and address, indicating too surely the real repression going on within of much that is lovable and admirable in a woman ... who does not know the shudder which a sensitive, highly wrought, fastidious man or woman speaks of those whose persons are continually before the world, whose names are bandied about, whose principles are discussed in half the drawing-rooms of London? that dreadful woman is the mildest term applied to them.

Nevertheless in her dress and even, perhaps, to some degree in her manners and opinions, the strong-minded woman was eventually to win the day. By the end of the 19th century, Charles Dana Gibson's sweet American girl graduates, walking beside their handsome male counterparts and making charmingly foolish remarks, were to appear wearing tightly belted masculine shirts, stiff collars and plain ties with boaters tilted on bewitchingly unruly curls. [47, 55] But side by side with this young charmer, with her tennis and her bicycling breeches, there still survived, at least in *Punch*, the pince-nez'd woman with drawn features who wore her mannish clothing with what looks, today, like grim despair [24]. Phil May was only one of the artists who drew her, strap-hanging in an omnibus and mocked at by a cloth-capped male who tells her that if she believes in women's rights she can stand up for them.

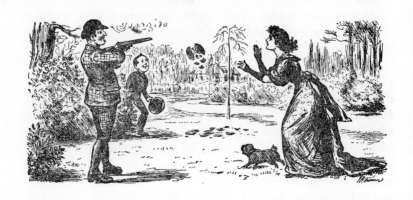

5

The Early 'Eighties

By the end of the 1870s there can have been few middle-class English women who could not read the language of contemporary dress, at least to the extent of recognising what was indubitably high-fashion, what had been labelled 'Pre-Raphaelite', what was meant by 'strong-minded' and what doctors and reformers asked for when they clamoured for reform. The majority of women struggled along of course in the wake of conventional fashion, keeping their toes as near to the heels of Paris as they, or their husbands' incomes, could manage.

There was a short interval at the end of the 'seventies and

the beginning of the 'eighties (the moment admired by Mrs Haweis) when those who followed high-fashion wore neither crinolettes nor bustles. Preceded, or followed by, this new straight dress which covered her like a sheath, a new ideal woman appeared who no longer looked her best in profile. It was, indeed, only from the front that this revised design for a woman could be understood, and then only when, upright and still, she stood with her head a little on one side so that her body achieved its balance by assuming a gentle curve from chin to toe, knees together, the whole weight resting on one foot while the other, set a little apart, touched the ground only with the toe. This new beauty had abandoned the Venus of Milos for the Venus of Botticelli. [18]

Probably unconscious of Walter Pater's ecstatic eloquence when he wrote his famous essay on Botticelli in 1872, most people who recognised that something had changed the look of fashionable women at the end of the 'seventies thought that they had become mediaeval. They were not altogether wrong for the newly admired Italian primitives did, in the contemporary mind, include Botticelli and were considered mediaeval. For a brief moment even the fashion-conscious Renoir tilted the head of a quite unmediaeval Parisian girl and painted her frontally with knees together, swathed in the newest Paris thing. [15] In this he was no more sensitive than the *haute couture* itself nor the rest of his fellow-painters in the *école de Paris* at catching a glimpse of the new ideas that were penetrating the air.

The woman of fashion who wore her sheath dress and held herself in the fashionable 'S' shape was of course usually unconscious that she was, like those with artistic taste, contributing to the prevailing mediaevalism or that while related to a 14th-century French Virgin she also looked like a lady in a Japanese print. These were characteristics she would have regarded as the province of the aesthetes. [20] It was W. S. Gilbert who publicised the shape in his new opera *Patience* which had its first production not as intended at the Savoy, which was not ready, but in the Strand at the Opera Comique in 1881. Gilbert knew that words appropriate to aesthetes were 'drooping', 'languid', and 'mediaeval', but failed, for all his perspicuity, to see that they also applied, though in a mild and disguised form, to the current orthodox fashion too, which certainly had a hint about it of the 'writhing maid, lithe limbed'.[1]

All the same, Gilbert saw a good deal. When he opposed his 'fleshly poet' (more Swinburne than Wilde, who had hardly begun to write poetry when *Patience* was produced) to a contingent of the Dragoon Guards, he gave one of his indignant female aesthetes – bowled over by the horror of their uniforms – the exclamation: 'Red and yellow! Primary colours! Oh, South Kensington!'[2] He also made her deplore the fact that red and yellow were not 'Early English' whereas cobwebby grey velvet with a tender bloom like cold gravy was. Bunthorne, the fleshly poet, pointed out that

> Though the Philistine may jostle, you will rank as an apostle in
> the high aesthetic band

> If you walk down Piccadilly with a poppy or a lily in your
> mediaeval hand.[3]

The mediaevalism was quite as important as the flower.

Even the Dragoons in *Patience* admitted at last that mediaeval art alone retained its zest. They realised that high aesthetic taste could not be bought ready-made like a pair of trousers, and that only Time would diffuse true views on mediaevalism. Yet they hoped that

> If you hold yourself like this
> And you hold yourself like that,[4]

you might, by assuming correctly writhing poses, win the girls. Having achieved their correctly aesthetic physical attitudes the Guards were rewarded by being called Botticellian and Fra Angelican.[5]

In fact Gilbert had little sympathy with the aesthetes, almost all of whom are de-aestheticised by the opera's end and have become what he describes as 'Every-day' young men and girls: the one exception, the fleshly poet, is left solitary with his flowers.

In October 1881, *Patience* was transferred from the Opera Comique to the new Savoy Theatre, built expressly to house the Gilbert and Sullivan operas. The new programme described *Patience* as the 'Celebrated Aesthetic Opera in Two Acts' and further stated that the entire auditorium was illuminated by Electric Light, 'by which the purity and coolness of the air' was preserved. The Swan incandescent lamps, continued the programme, emitted a soft yellow light and there was no unpleasant glare; in a few days, it was promised, this light would be applied also on the stage. The chorus had been increased, the opera newly mounted and dressed, and it is surprising to discover from the programme that the Aesthetic Dresses were designed by the author.

It was Lady Jane, the comic heavy aesthetic maiden who, faced with the red and gold uniforms of the Guards, had invoked the College of Art, exclaiming 'Oh, South Kensington!'. Mrs Haweis, however, would not have shared her faith. For while convinced that education would eventually develop good taste in everybody she was not sure how this could be achieved. Certainly not, in her view, through the art schools of South Kensington and Gower Street which '*taught* too much and *educated* too little'.

What, she wondered, could 'help us in at the Gate which is called beautiful to train up artisans and workmen to whom we may entrust whatsoever we want made fair?'[6]

After reading *Patience*, Mrs Haweis's language sounds dangerously Gilbertian. She certainly belonged to the social group that had inspired him; and even three years before *Patience* was produced she had been prepared to formulate at least some rules that would ensure good taste in dress. Colours, she thought, should not be too pure, a trap which manufacturers had fallen into, urged on by the public's vulgar craving for gaudiness. Colours faded by age were more beautiful than in their pristine freshness, and hence the old-fashioned blue which had a dash of yellow in it was preferable, even though it should look sadly faded, to fashionable blues.

On the design of dress Mrs Haweis was equally confident:

> As for the skirt ... it must partake of the character of the bodice – that is to say, if the bodice be cut tightly and formally to the figure, the skirt should be so. For instance, none but a plain skirt without a single plait, can properly go with a tight bodice. But if the bodice be full at the waist the skirt must contain plaits – for this form must signify a full and folded garment closed to the waist with a girdle. Nothing could be worst taste than to wear a loose bodice such as a Garibaldi, with a tight gored skirt ... It at once betrays that the skirt and bodice do not belong to each other, are not cut together or, as artists say, 'Not all painted with the same palette'.[7]

Mrs Haweis was no innovator but she was a sensitive barometer. Consciously or not she was describing the two contrasting fashions current at the time of writing. The paragraph quoted above comes from her book *The Art of Beauty*, published in 1878 and presumably written, therefore, in 1877, the year when the crinolette with its back projection was replaced by the 'princess' line which, while fitting the body closely, poured down from shoulder to foot with no three-dimensional break. Seen from the front the suggestion of the nude through the dense outer-sheath of this dress was a daring feature and a composition which had not been used since the beginning of the 15th century, when it was disappearing after a long innings. So W. S. Gilbert was not altogether wrong in his choice of the mediaeval hand as a symbol that fitted the moment.

The deference with which Mrs Haweis was treated not only as her books appeared, one following the other rapidly at the end of the 'seventies, but also in the half-decade that followed seems, today, surprising. Unless she was speaking of dress itself she always trod cautiously and qualified her assertions with a 'to some extent'. Speaking of what she called 'Imbecile Ornament', she ventured on saying:

> Probably nothing that is not useful is in any high sense beautiful,[8]

thereby linking herself with those who were sensitive enough to recognise the 'high sense' in a quality or emotion. As Miss Lonsdale was soon to point out in writing of the platform woman, the 'fastidious' and 'highly wrought' should be protected from outrages to their feelings.

Mrs Haweis admitted the significance of the Greeks: indeed in her period she could hardly have done otherwise; but she considered that an attempt to imitate them was not practicable. In her *Art of Dress* of 1879 she went so far as to call Greek dress

> the most perfect form of known costume . . . the human body is not necessarily a shocking thing . . . But what was harmless to the Greeks would be impossible to Nations who have lost to a great extent the simple instinct of natural beauty, whilst they have grown abnormally self-conscious and reflective.[9]

She furthermore considered the simple chyton, pretty as it was, too difficult to wear to please those not young and 'finely-moulded' and too monotonous to please everybody. She also thought that although the English type was robust and lovely, the race was too mixed to endure one costume. Of her two ideal types of dress, the close-fitting and the full, it was the latter, the dress gathered into folds down both the bodice and the skirt and held by a girdle, that corresponded to what was generally held to be and what she herself had described in her articles in the *Queen* as PreRaphaelite dress.

Respected as she was in her own day, Mrs Haweis's view of the period was, in reality, a narrow and superficial one for, from the beginning to the end of the decade, the 1880s represented the *grande époque* in 19th-century reform, by no means limited to the design of dress. In spite of the apprehensions of its opponents, the Reform Bill itself had produced no evil results. Following it both political parties committed themselves with increasing momentum to introduce further measures which would improve the lot of the people of England; to engineer the happiness and well-being of every deserving Englishman was seen to be, given time, a practical proposition and, in such an atmosphere, it seemed to most people that those who were undeserving would soon cease to be so.

To many of those who had lived through the 1880s and looked back on them from the end of the 19th century, they seemed to be particularly marked by an improvement in public taste. Writing on the literature of the period, H. D. Traill, for instance, regarded the 'eighties as a decade which saw both the sharp decline in popularity of the miserably third-rate Martin Tupper and the wide-spread recognition of Algernon Swinburne not only as a first-rate poet but as a major influence on the younger poets of the rising generation.[10] Reviewing, from the turn of the century, the fine arts of the 1880s, F. G. Stephens saw Millais, Rossetti, and Whistler as the giants of the period with Lord Leighton and Burne-Jones as admirable runners-up. Stephens' opinion of Whistler is striking, especially from one who also saw the earlier importance of Ruskin. He hailed Whistler as a fine and original artist and a rare colourist, and regarded it as his misfortune rather than his fault that he had been saddled with 'so-called Impressionism' which, artistically speaking, was his 'illegitimate offspring'. Even so, he continued, 'neither the fads and vagaries of the New English Art Club . . . nor the crude and audacious vulgarities of MM Degas and Manet' ought to be fathered on him.[11]

Writing on the decorative arts, May Morris too noticed that there had been a long-overdue improvement in public taste in the 'eighties. Although she recognised that by then the Pre-Raphaelite movement itself was long dead, she regarded its influence as having, if anything, grown stronger. Both the 'enormities of the Great Exhibition of 1851' and the 'monumental dulness of that of 1862' were, May Morris declared, forgotten, and side by side with the revolution in domestic design on which William Morris (her father) and his associates were working, a new inspiration had appeared in the East as a result of the break-up of the Japanese feudal republic in 1868.

With the consequent opening of her frontiers there arrived on the European market first a trickle and by the 'eighties a steady flow of Japanese treasures ranging from precious objects from private collections, some of them of great antiquity, to cheap but startlingly attractive contemporary prints, all of which opened the eyes of both artists and the public to new artistic possibilities. Moreover they were objects which seemed all the better for having nothing in common with the lush exuberance of the middle of the 19th century, the moment which represented in the eyes of the 'eighties, the nadir of taste.[12]

Both F. G. Stephens and May Morris, the first reviewing the fine arts of the 'eighties and the second the applied arts, agreed that Walter Crane, though still at an early stage in his career, had played a considerable part in the improvement of public taste.

Such assessments may not coincide with ours today nor, exactly, with the opinion that the 'eighties held of their own artistic scene, but Traill was probably right in his view that while neither Tennyson nor Browning (whose genius the public had been slow to recognise) could halt the 'many-sided prostration before the commonplace, ... the sudden and startling apparition of Mr Swinburne' was able to achieve this miracle.[13]

Both Swinburne and Whistler had, of course, established the personal style by which each was to be recognised long before 1880, but according to Traill and Stephens the 'eighties saw their significance appreciated by their contemporaries.

The charge of the 'prostration before the commonplace' on the part of the 1850s and 1860s was probably justified: a magazine manifestly designed to be read by fairly intelligent people had published, in 1868, an article with the title Useful Mediocrity, which declared that 'we already have a good stock of first-rate art for those who can enjoy it; let us have some creditable mediocrity for persons of lesser education or natural capacity'[14] – a plea that could have been put forward nowhere in the 1880s when the aim of all serious men and women was to raise the taste of people of all classes by means of unremitting education and never to express a wish for anything but the best in any of the creative arts.

What apparently none of the critics writing in the 'nineties and looking back to the 'eighties noticed (or if they did they chose to ignore it) was the continuing passionate admiration for the arts and the lives of the ancient Greeks which remained, although only one, an important aspect of taste. Incidents, real or imaginary, from classical Greece, and women in Grecian draperies were, however, still providing subjects for Leighton, Poynter, and even occasionally for Watts; and heroines in fiction continued to resemble heroines of the Golden Age in their physique. George Meredith's *Diana of the Crossways* must have been written in 1883 (it appeared serialised in the *Fortnightly* in 1884 and in stiff covers 'greatly enlarged' in 1885), thirteen years after Disraeli's *Lothair*; but Meredith's Diana Warwick's looks were still those of Disraeli's Theodora Campain: 'Mrs Warwick is "quite Grecian". She might pose for a statue'.[15] This is emphasised by the fact that when he described the girl whom he presented as a very indifferent second to the ravishing Diana, Meredith painted an out-moded beauty; one who, thirty years earlier, Dickens would certainly have chosen for a heroine but who was no longer acceptable in the 'eighties. Constance 'was white from head to foot; a symbol of purity. Judging from her look and her reputation ... the man was justly mated with a devious filmy sentimentalist'.[16] Like Theodora Campian, Diana Warwick was an active not a passive heroine.

Mrs Campian, an early specimen of post-Mill heroine – *Lothair* was published in 1870 – had plotted, fought, and died for the liberation of Italy. She had been dangerous to her admirers, including Lothair who fell under her spell, and had been prepared to sacrifice them to the Cause. Meredith's Diana Warwick, as witty and intelligent as she was lovely, was dangerous only to those too coarse-grained to apprehend her essential innocence; a later example of the post-Mill woman, she discussed the minutiae of the Corn Laws with Ministers of State, refreshing them after long hours in the Commons or Lords and, at the same time, providing them with telling points for the following days' debates. She not only served but valued the best wines, her French chef was superb, and her house decorated, naturally, with treasures from the Orient. She did not, however, herself lead campaigns – the high hopes of the end of the 'sixties had receded as far as women in the field of politics were concerned.

To be coarse-grained was inexcusable in the 'eighties. It was during the serial appearance of *Diana of the Crossways* in the *Fortnightly Review* that the same journal published Margaret Lonsdale's attack on the platform woman, expressing the fear that she might appear 'dreadful' to men and women who were, 'sensitive, highly-wrought, fastidious'. Brilliant as she was, Meredith's Diana Warwick was never allowed to speak from a platform, and when she was forced to earn her living by writing novels, they appeared under a pseudonym; she was admired by men and women alike, and her only enemies were those too obtuse to understand her sparkling sallies – the insensitive. Dazzling enough to have succeeded in any profession or office, she never attempted to edge herself into either and she was, one gathers, only too glad to lay down her pen when she was relieved of financial worries. Had she been created fifteen years earlier or five years later, at the end of the 'eighties, she would probably not have feared the limelight.

Meredith never indulged in long descriptions of dress. He mentions Diana's clothing only once but his brief account of her appearance, early one morning on a mountain-side near Lugano, is enough to establish both her taste and his own understanding of the current language of dress. She is gathering purple meadow crocuses, themselves a part of the picture of Diana.

> She was dressed in some texture of the hue of lavender. A violet scarf loosely knotted over the bosom opened on her throat. The loop of her black hair curved under a hat of gray beaver ... some sweet wild cyclamen flowers were at her breast.[17]

This comes very near to a Whistler 'Harmony in Violet and Grey'.

Although only a woman sensitive to the artistic taste of the time would have chosen to look like that in 1883, there were evidently enough of her kind for another journal, the *Nineteenth Century*, to consider that the whole question of the design of women's dress would be of interest to its readers, for the following year they published a long article by G. F. Watts with the title *On Taste in Dress*.

Watts approached the subject with considerably more hesitation than Mrs Haweis had done – he warmed to it later – for he saw that good taste in female dress was, to a great extent, a matter of opinion. Furthermore, unlike most of his contemporaries he felt that

The waywardness of feminine fashion is not a subject for puritanical objection; the changeableness affords occupation for many, and variety is a better thing than monotony ...
The varieties and vagaries of fashion are the natural outcome of society, leisure and wealth. The sober thinker will not condemn or discourage them.[18]

With a sort of grandiose humility mixed with some pompous arrogance, Watts, in his long article, felt his way through the complexities of the subject of women's dress; among many other points he decided that in the midst of the changing fashions of the 19th-century one feature appeared to be permanent – the small waist – and this he deplored. In seeing that 'a small waist is only pretty when harmonising with youthfulness and general slightness',[19] he probably put his finger on the reason for its long popularity in the 19th century: it was a symbol of youth in a period of very tightly restrictive dress. If he hesitated to present a concrete picture of a dress that would be in good taste, Watts was, nevertheless, prepared to define bad taste as a violation of established principles, thinking that 'the Greek canons of human proportion may be taken as established into law',[20] – although he recognised only too well that the Greek canon of human proportion, particularly the relationship of the size of the head to the height of the body, was rarely to be found in real life. By the standards of Greek sculpture most heads were too large, and when, therefore, a small head could be found it was always, he pointed out, considered a great beauty. From this he argued that any fashion which enlarged the appearance of the head by 'piling up enormous masses of hair, mostly or always false', must be in bad taste.[21]

As so often happens when matters of taste are discussed, at the moment when Watts was propounding his law, the fashion for enlarging the head with piled-up masses of hair had recently gone out, to be replaced by a small neat hairdressing. There must naturally have been a great many women who were slow to relinquish the former style; and since these were more likely to have included elderly and conservative than young and therefore more attractive women, their presence would have served to emphasise Watts's argument. Almost venomously he continued:

> To outweigh the upright human figure with an immense quantity of hair massed into a solid lump is to distort that fitness without which there is no harmony or beauty.[22]

The puffed-out chignon of the 'seventies had not, of course, been thought of at the time as a solid lump and, when it was fashionable, it had been balanced by a figure greatly enlarged by a crinolette and a train. Watts's 'upright human figure' was, in itself, a relatively new conception which had succeeded the Grecian bend.

In his appreciation of the small head, Watts carried his sensitivity to current fashion further by declaring that bonnets made of 'dense' materials should be small and that when large hats were worn these should be made of light and airy materials. Among the most fashionable circles of the early 'eighties, bonnets were the required type of formal head-dress and were at their tiniest; large hats, considered to be informal, were worn only in high summer when they would, in any case, have been unlikely to be 'dense'. Meredith's Diana Warwick could have been forgiven for wearing a grey beaver hat, certainly dense, since she was, at the time, travelling.

Watts regarded a fringe of hair across the forehead as pretty and acceptable in youth but he thought it should be clearly understood that it concealed one of humanity's most beautiful features – the spring and growth of the hair on the forehead. Apart from the evil of wearing false hair, however, the most objectionable practice in his view would be to part the hair on one side since this disturbed the balance:

> The two sides of all organic structures always corresponding even in what is purely ornamental.[23]

In the 1880s he would not have been in danger of finding many heads on which the hair was parted at the side.

Where the design of dress itself was concerned, Watts went further than contemporary critics of fashion. He agreed with them that shapes, particularly protuberances, which produced a distorted impression of the human body were bad. He also saw the human neck, rising like a stem or column from square shoulders, as a beauty possessed by mankind alone among the animals; therefore, because they concealed it, he condemned the wearing of collars by both men and women. Crinolines and dresses with long trains he considered 'extravagant in form but selfish in disregard of the convenience of others; selfishness cannot be good taste'.[24] Excessive tightness, too, was undesirable. Tight sleeves made the arms look like sausages; hands squeezed into gloves too small for them rendered them useless – incapable, that is to say, of clasping the hand of another with the full fervour of friendship or pulling a child out of danger. [31] The Greeks, he pointed out, had rejected smallness of hand; proportion and fineness were their ruling principles. And Watts naturally devoted a good deal of space to the condemnation of stays and corsets which, by constricting the torso, made it look like a 'length of pipe'.

> General amplitude is indeed far from ungracious, but on the contrary carries a dignity that is pleasant to look upon; but short violent curves are eminently ugly.[25]

Short violent curves were inevitably produced by those women who, deploring a gracious amplitude of figure, compressed their waists and ribs by means of a tight corset.

All this is, of course, Watts the painter writing, and in the period of the statuesque beauty, the type of woman who had, for more than a decade, been glorified in fiction as well as in his own paintings and in those of most of his contemporaries. Though she was never abandoned by Watts, there were painters – Whistler, for instance – who in the 'eighties felt that she was on the way out. It was not easy to reconcile figures of the proportions of those on the Parthenon pediment with the taste for Early English, and although most of Watts's contemporaries agreed, no doubt, that short violent curves were ugly (they had lately been noticeably absent from the *haute couture*) there were probably some, Walter Crane among them perhaps, who did not. Sandwiched between the luxuriant Watteau toilette and the sharp precise fashions of the middle 'eighties, the Botticellian line was permitted only a short moment of life by Parisian designers; the crinolette was already returning when Watts's article appeared and, in its new form, was to depend largely on short violent curves.

Discussing colour and texture, which he did only very briefly in his article on Taste in Dress, it was Watts the adorer of the later Venetians who spoke (most of his fellow painters would have thought of colour differently):

Quantity of material should govern form . . . so the closely-fitting cuirasse, splendid in maroon velvet or other noble textures and colours, would not look so well in simple colourless materials.[26]

Cultivated critics of the 'eighties were not agreed on the question of colour. Some of them admired the cool blues and greyish greens of Burne-Jones and the veiled harmonies of Whistler, while others found these 'muddy' and preferred small precise areas of brighter colour used in a mediaeval way. Watts's Venetian taste did not fall into either category and was not, at the time, influential.

Reviewing an exhibition at the *avant garde* Grosvenor Gallery in May 1884, the critic of the *Daily News* found that

in a dim hall, where the uncertain light was too yellow for
slate colour and too grey for mud, a shivering ghostly train
of critics were busy with their tasks. They looked like men
condemned in some aesthetic inferno, to puzzle forever over
pictures without colour or meaning.[27]

Since this was written three years after the Savoy Theatre had
boasted of the soft yellow glow of its new electric lighting, it
sounds very conservative, but the critic of the *Daily News* did
find one at least among the paintings to approve, though he
considered it difficult to discuss from the point of view of
colour. This painting was Burne-Jones's huge *King Cophetua
and the Beggar Maid*, exhibited for the first time: 'Words fail us
to depict the blending and shifting hues of his dress', a problem
he solved by quoting Ruskin's already hackneyed 'colours that
find no name this side of heaven'.[28]

He advised his fellow critics to follow his example and search
their Ruskins for terms in which to express their feelings.
Although he actually admired the picture's colour and found
its subject acceptable, the critic of the *Daily News* was unable to
account for the Maid's dreary and mystically distressed facial
expression, for, he said, 'if ever there was a lucky girl it was the
beggar's daughter'.[29] an opinion that would not have been
voiced, surely, by one more highly wrought and fastidious. It
seems strange, too, that three years after the production of
Patience art critics were still thinking of the Grosvenor Gallery
in terms that Gilbert would have used to describe the milieu of
Reginald Bunthorn. Colour juxtapositions and combinations of
the kind variously used by Burne-Jones and Whistler had
certainly been accepted and imitated in the early 'eighties by
women who wore artistic dress, but they must also have
permeated, though unrecognised for what they were, the world
of the *haute couture*; in 1884 mutations of one subdued colour
were constantly used together in fashionable dress. The clothes
of ladies visiting the private views during the month that King
Cophetua was exhibited at the Grosvenor Gallery were
especially chosen as the subject of an article by the fashion
columnist of the *Daily News*. The private views were important

and attended by everybody of social or artistic significance. At them could be found 'the triumphs of Elise and Redfern down to the nondescript garb of maidens who call themselves "intense", and who walk about with a flower held in the listless fingers of one hand'.[30] Although the fashion writers were manifestly irritated by innovations and eccentricities, they had to be noticed.

The mediaeval hand, it appears, still fingered its flowers in public but the journalist who covered the fashions at the private views for the *Daily News* could surely have done better by searching Ruskin or even Gilbert for an adjective more appropriate than 'nondescript' to identify artistic dress in 1884, though it might have been too much to expect a daily paper to notice that even the grand creations of the *haute couture* reflected the Grosvenor Gallery taste. In preferring 'mushroom colours' to Watts's 'noble maroon' Paris designers had already adjusted themselves to the new artistic scene. Among the many toilettes in mushroom colours, one was described as being worn with a bonnet to match, in which 'a bunch of kingcups offered the only relief from the pale fawn tints'; and this is typical of many colour-combinations that were described. The wearer of the kingcups, we are told, 'jostled a Burne-Jonesian girl in a long dark red silk mantle with a night-cap to match'.[31] In the same article the author continued by longing for an Act of Parliament to frame a sumptuary law which would prohibit the wearing of muddy colours by those whose complexions were of the same hue.

A month later the *Daily News* included among its advertisements one which recommended 'Nonpareil' velveteen for 'its great depth of pile which absorbed all dazzling light and lent a gentle subdued and ladylike aspect'[32] to those who wore it. And who were they? W. S. Gilbert could surely have answered, for it was his Lady Jane who sighed for Dragoon Guards wearing

cobwebby grey velvet, with a tender bloom like cold gravy which, made Florentine fourteenth-century, trimmed with Venetian leather and Spanish altar-lace, and surmounted by something Japanese – would at least be Early English.[33]

With or without the inspiration of the Grosvenor Gallery and those who exhibited there, fashion in the early 'eighties had turned decisively away from the brilliant colours that had emerged in rapid succession from chemical laboratories of the 'sixties and 'seventies to be snatched up by all fashionable women of the time. The revulsion was normal, it is the attention devoted by the press to the new subdued colours which is interesting. Writing of a distinguished gathering a reporter to the *Pall Mall Gazette* of May 4th 1884 observed:

> Mr Oscar Wilde discoursed in his free and easy way ... In critical vein Mr Wilde shook his shorn and curling locks, and, fanning himself with an expensive sage-green silk pocket handkerchief ... lowered his slim form gracefully into the bosom of a yielding couch.[34]

Not only was sage green, especially in silk, a Burne-Jonesian tint but the *Pall Mall Gazette's* reporter had been acute enough to know that it was worth recording when used by Oscar Wilde. Two months later even the fashion representative of the *Daily News* had accepted the fact that the best-dressed woman was easily identified: 'the colours she wears delight the eye, there are no violent contrasts, no crude tints, all is soft and harmonious',[35] which was what George Meredith had understood so well when, at almost precisely the same moment, he had chosen to dress his Diana Warwick in a texture 'of the hue of lavender', giving her a bunch of wild cyclamen in her bosom and knotting a violet scarf loosely round her neck.

In 1881, the year of the production of *Patience*, W. P. Frith, who would certainly not have been rated by his contemporaries as a sensitive artist in the new aesthetic sense, decided, apparently quite independently of Gilbert's libretto, to immortalise those who wore artistic dress in a painting of the Private View at the Royal Academy [29]. Of his motives for doing so there can be no doubt, for in the second volume of his autobiography, which was published in 1887, he mentioned the painting and recollected:

Seven years ago certain ladies delighted to display themselves
at public gatherings in what are called aesthetic dresses; in
some cases the dresses are pretty enough, in others they
seem to rival each other in ugliness of form and oddity of
colour. They were – and still are I believe – preachers of
aestheticism in dress ... Beyond the desire of recording for
posterity the aesthetic craze as regards dress, I wished to hit
the folly of listening to self-elected critics in matters of taste
whether in dress or art.[36]

There is a not altogether surprising tinge of bitterness in
Frith's determination to hit 'self-elected critics', for by 1881 he
was himself a back number whose pictures of the 'fifties and
'sixties had long been out of fashion. Frith had always been a
painter of crowds and in his *Private View* he was faithful to his
old theme though he could no longer handle it with the same
ease. Among the famous and the fashionable in his picture,
one of the self-elected was, presumably, Oscar Wilde who is
evidently commenting on the paintings on the walls, catalogue
in hand and surrounded by an admiring group; but in the
account of the painting that Frith included in his memoirs of
six years later he did not mention Wilde by name though he
did explain that 'on the left of the composition is a family of
pure aesthetes absorbed in affected study of the pictures ...
Mr Browning talks to an aesthetic lady whose draped back
affords a chance of showing that view of the costume'.[37]
In Frith's painting the dress of the pure aesthetes follows the
principles pronounced by Mrs Haweis. The lady and her child
on the left (regarded with amusement by Trollope who is
called by Frith a 'homely figure') wear dresses with folds in the
bodice which continue below the waist-belt down the skirt.
The lady's dress, which is orange, is lifted by a very casual
arrangement of drapery to show a white petticoat beneath. Her
companion, nearer the centre, wears Mrs Haweis's other type,
a dress with no folds at all. Its colour is olive green with a
yellow trimming, and a yellow sunflower is tucked into the
front of her bodice. This, presumably, is Frith's 'pure aesthete
absorbed in affected study of the pictures', but to us today her

dress, far from looking abnormal, seems hardly different in conception from the dress, which is not artistic, worn by Lady Lonsdale who sits in the centre of the painting talking to Leighton who is standing beside her. Although to us, however, the difference between the two is difficult to discern, the combination of olive green with yellow (which must have appeared ugly to Frith) and the failure to produce two violently concave curves at the waist, mark the dress worn by the lady of the sunflower as artistic.

The behaviour of all these artistic ladies, to judge from Frith's view of them, is very normal. They do not writhe, neither do they droop; Oscar Wilde's hand is nicely painted but scarcely mediaeval. On his right stands a lady who wears the most spectacular among the artistic dresses: it is pink, a long drapery flows down from the neck at the back and lies on the ground in an ample train. The little group who listen with evident respect to the exposition of Oscar Wilde is observed with interest by two or three men on the right, among them W. S. Gilbert whose definitely unaesthetic eye is fixed on the artistic dress of the lady in pink. Since the programme of *Patience* informs us that for the opening at the Savoy in October 1881, the year of Frith's picture, the aesthetic dresses were newly designed and by the author, Frith's placing of Gilbert in his painting may have been intentional.

The lady particularly mentioned by Frith as showing the back of an aesthetic dress and as talking to Robert Browning, stands on the spectator's left, wearing bluish-green. Hers is, probably, the truest version of PreRaphaelite dress as it survived in 1881.

Frith's fascinating documentary painting makes it clear that there was no social division between those who wore artistic dresses in the early 'eighties and those who did not. It also shows that in high society there was a good deal of it about. But the strong-minded woman, is nowhere to be seen – she was a pariah in society, undignified and uncomfortable to recollect, a view of her that was, perhaps, one of the triumphs of the aestheticians.

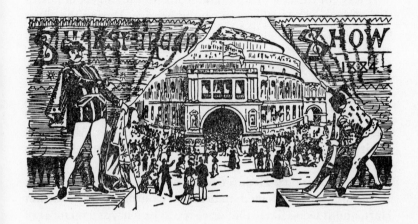

6

Sanitarians and Woolleners

Although for more than a century doctors had been worried about the unhealthiness of successive fashions in dress, no serious attempt had been made to convince the public that, provided they were willing to ignore current canons of beauty, designers could produce clothing that was really sanitary. The proof came in 1884 when the International Health Exhibition in London included an important section on hygienic dress.

The International Health Exhibition was an event of considerable significance which has been neglected by later social historians. It covered a very large area in Kensington which, from the back of the Natural History Museum, was bounded on the east by what is now the Exhibition Road and took in, on the north, the Albert Hall.

It was not the first exhibition devoted to the subject of health though it was by far the most comprehensive. During the 1870s exhibitions had been held in connection with annual congresses of the Social Science Association at Leeds, Norwich, Glasgow, Liverpool and Brighton; and in 1883 the first exhibition to deal exclusively with health was organised by the National Health Society and held, according to the British Medical Journal, in a 'large iron building in Knightsbridge since known as Humphrey's Hall'. The Smoke Abatement Institute had already arranged an exhibition in South Kensington in 1881.

Both the National Health Society and the Smoke Abatement Institute were conducted under the chairmanship of Ernest Hart, and it seems likely that since it was he who, as a member of the Executive Committee, delivered the closing speech when the International Health Exhibition of 1884 finally closed its doors, the whole enterprise had come into being as the result of his efforts.

Apart from the Albert Hall the actual buildings on the extensive Kensington site had already been occupied the previous year by an International Fisheries Exhibition at the closing of which, in October 1883, the Prince of Wales had announced his intention of organising a Health Exhibition to be held on the same spot the following year. It would, said His Royal Highness, be presented on a great scale and under his personal presidency.

> This exhibition is intended to illustrate the most advanced knowledge in respect to the applications of modern science and improved sanitary practice to the dwelling and its curtilage and to food and dress. . . . Such a display is especially opportune at the present moment when health questions are assuming a position of primary importance in the policy of Governments and in ministerial functions, as well as in the private duty of individuals . . . . it will be organised so as to embrace and bring into prominence illustrations of all that

must affect the welfare of the people, not forgetting the poorer classes.

The exhibition was to include the home, food and sanitation in every walk of life; and also dress, which,

in its relation to hygiene, climate and to the various purposes in industrial occupations, in historic retrospection, will afford an opportunity for illustration of an artistic and useful character.

It is clear, therefore, that in the enthusiasm for hygiene, art could not be excluded although attempts to combine the two were to lead to difficulties.

The main purpose of the International Health Exhibition was to awaken the people of England to the importance of healthy living in every aspect of their lives but in the event it included many less serious delights such as Chinese and Japanese restaurants where oriental cooking could be enjoyed.

On January 1st 1884, *The Times* printed an advertisement from C. B. Pare & Co, Exhibition Contractors, offering to receive exhibits, and on January 11th a notice by the Duke of Buckingham and Chandos, Chairman of the Executive Committee of the International Health Exhibition, stipulated that all goods intended for display must be in their places by May 1st. On May 1st *The Times* carried an advertisement which stated that the Patron of the exhibition was H.M. the Queen and that it would be opened on Thursday, May 8th. Admission to the opening ceremony would be by season ticket. The Exhibition would remain open from 10 a.m. to 11.30 p.m. Season tickets would cost a guinea and single admission one shilling, except on Wednesdays when it would be half-a-crown.

The Prince of Wales had consented to open the Exhibition, but on the opening day itself a leader in *The Times* explained that owing to the unexpected death of his younger brother, the Duke of Albany, the opening ceremony would be performed by the Duke of Cambridge, though the Prince would remain acting President.

During the days that followed the opening the Exhibition received a great deal of attention from the Press. A leader in *The Times* on the opening day, after explaining that a block of Old London had been contributed by the generosity of the City Guilds (*The Illustrated London News* carried illustrations of some of the buildings), pointed out that although mediaeval revivalists would be sure to put the pleasant side of their period uppermost

> modern Sanitarians on their part are endowed with a very dissimilar spirit of brutal candour . . . Under the Plantagenets and Tudors simplicity on sanitary matters doubtless was overdone, still Englishmen existed and, at all events in Cheapside, in a fair degree of comfort. The Science of Health threatens now to go to the opposite extreme and bury life under the resources for protecting it.[1]

Throughout the summer special attractions were mounted as a part of the Exhibition. [33] Inside the arena of the Albert Hall, for instance, a large area was used for a 'Shakespearean Show' [Headpiece to chapter 6 and no. 34] in aid of the Chelsea Hospital for Women, and special sections included exhibits on health in China and in India. Since, however, the fundamental aim was to improve conditions in English domestic and industrial life, the greater part was naturally devoted to drainage, ventilation and anti-pollution schemes which the public were encouraged to examine along with other more titillating innovations.

The International Health Exhibition, which soon became affectionately known as the Healtheries, was an immense success and prolonged far beyond its original closing date at the beginning of August. On August 1st, indeed, a further advertisement in *The Times* (by then the advertisements of exhibitors ran to two columns) insisted that applications to exhibit at the I.H.E. must be received before October 1st.

The area devoted to dress occupied a large part of the Grand Circle in the Albert Hall [32] which was arranged to display the various classes into which the sub-committee had decided to divide the subject:

The History of Dress, National Costume etc.
Waterproof clothing, India rubber, gutta percha etc.
Furs, skins and feathers – Dress for extreme climates etc.
Dress for sport, hunting suits etc.
Life saving dress, divers' dress, fireproof dress.
Publications and literature related to Group 2; patterns, statistics, diagrams and models.
Machines and appliances for the preparation of articles under group 2.

Furthermore, 'The sub-committee would suggest that to the classes named in this group another class should be added dealing with the comparative value of different dress materials as articles of clothing'.[2]

The history of clothing took the form of reconstructions of past fashions mounted on full-size wax models designed by Madame Tussaud and arranged chronologically. This exhibit was extremely popular especially since 'good' and 'bad' periods could be compared. Any period that had extended the skirt by means of understructures automatically came into the category 'bad', and it was generally agreed that the dress of the reign of Edward I was the most beautiful.

Naturally the search for beauty was not the aim of the Exhibition; in every comment on the show the importance of hygiene was stressed. Among the articles in *The Times* on the days that followed the opening, a column on May 9th was devoted to the section of Dress which had been arranged under the direction of the Hon. Lewis Wingfield. *The Times* noted that the 'chronological display gave an opportunity for a comparative study of civilian dress in its bearings on hygiene at different periods in the nation's growth';[3] and this was also the theme of a lecture given on this section of the Exhibition by E. W. Godwin, which was later issued as one of the pamphlets printed in connection with the I.H.E.

Godwin had opened his lecture by saying:

As Architecture is the art and science of building, so Dress is the art and science of clothing. To construct and decorate a covering for the human body that shall be beautiful and healthy is as important as to build a shelter for it when so covered that shall be beautiful and healthy. Where art is a living reality with peoples, their costumes will be the first to declare it; and quite the surest sign of the hollowness of modern art – pretentiousness – is, that our dress remains a limbeck not reflecting anything, be our homes fashioned like that of the architecture of the time of Sophocles or Virgil, of Beowulf or Chaucer, of Shakespeare or Goldsmith . . . to breathe in an atmosphere where the sunbeam throbs with art, and the rain is woven with sanitation, are, perhaps, possible only in Utopia . . . Science and art must walk hand in hand if life is to be worth living. Beauty without health is incomplete. Health can never be perfect so long as your eye is troubled with ugliness.[4]

After Godwin, the prose and the theories of William Morris, who contributed a lecture on textiles (also printed as a pamphlet), are simple and down to earth but it was Godwin who had emphasised the dilemma of the time – the problem of equating beauty and health in concrete terms. Godwin saw that one thing was quite clear:

in the climate of transpontine Europe the old classic dress cannot be revived. Indeed, except on a substratum warm and reasonably tight-fitting, such as is provided by the bifurcated garment known as *combinations*, the characteristic beauties of classic dress cannot be realised.[5]

The bifurcated garment, whether worn outside or beneath, was to be a controversial issue during the rest of the 'eighties.

Apart from the chronological display of fashions of the past, among the classes into which the section devoted to Dress was divided was one consisting of a collection of chemicals used to make muslins and other light fabrics non-inflammable and in the same class chemical dyes which were poisonous were contrasted with safe natural dyes. An exhibit of knitted and woven woollen goods dyed with innocuous dyes specially im-

ported from India was shown too, but even these apparently
safe colourings were by no means accepted by all theorists on
the subject of dress. Among the rough home-spun friezes and
the hand-knitted socks and stockings made in Britain was a
novelty advocated by many who believed in healthy dress –
socks and stockings hand-knitted in wool and made like gloves
so that each toe was covered separately [38]. Obviously, these
could be worn only with roomy square-toed shoes or boots, but
since these, too, were shown and recommended in the exhibition's section on Dress, the only problem that remained was
the difficulty of seeing that they were beautiful. Aesthetes
considered that shoes with high heels and pointed toes were
ugly, but they found flat square-toed shoes hard to accept.
Sandals were preferable, but since an important part of the
philosophy of those who supported hygienic dress was that
the body should be completely covered by a layer of wool,
sandals could only be permissible if worn over woollen stockings. The stockings with divided toes did, however, have the
advantage of allowing their wearers to adopt sandals on the
oriental pattern which had a strap between the big toe and its
neighbour.

All these points were thoroughly discussed in the press including the *Lancet* and the *British Medical Journal*. The former called
attention to the fact that on the opening day among those at the
foot of the royal dais 'was Edwin Chadwick C.B. wearing a suit
of sanitary woollen clothing as devised by Dr Jaeger'.[6] [37] Dr
Jaeger, who will be discussed later, was an exhibitor in the
section on Dress. *The Times* reported that of all the departments
of the Health Exhibition, next to food, dress attracted most
attention. The historical section was popular but the crowds
really thronged along the opposite corridor where 'one object
of curiosity is a garment which alone among 19th century
fashions, if the useful but hideous mackintosh be excepted,
has no prototype in the collections Mr Wingfield has reproduced from fashions of bygone times, namely, the divided
skirt'.[7]

Very popular too were women actually engaged in making
gloves and hand-made lace. The *Pall Mall Gazette*, which was

running a series on 'Women who Work', deplored the fact that at an exhibition devoted to health, such sweated labour should be on view, unless perhaps, it might be wise to call the attention of the public to the terrible drudgery involved in making these luxurious things.

Mrs Gladstone, who contributed an article to the *Daily News* in June, took as her subject health in the nursery, but remarked in passing that she had found the advice of Mr Godwin kindly and gravely sensible. The home was very thoroughly examined for any articles of furnishing that might be injurious to health and it was discovered that wall-paper of a nice bright green colour should be particularly condemned for it contained arsenic and, if used in the nursery, might be licked by the young.

The medical profession was, needless to say, enthusiastic about most of the ideas put forward in the Healtheries, and doctors were ready to be quoted in any publications that would give them space. On May 14th a leader in the *Daily News* referred to the views of Dr Zacharie, the well-known ortho-paedist, on the dangers of forcing children's feet into tight boots. Straight narrow soles, he said, were always dangerous and never beautiful. Wide soles and square toes might at first appear ugly but the eye soon accustomed itself to them. He then fell back on the favourite theme of the Greeks whose sculptors had rendered the winged feet of Mercury so beauti-fully. The *Daily News* thought that poets were in a large measure to blame for the unhealthy business. They were, from the sanitary point of view, a decidedly mischievous race: they admired small tapering waists which encouraged the agonies involved in attempting to 'crib cabin and confine excesses of adipose tissue'; and from Sir John Suckling down to the present Poet Laureate they sang the praises of fairy feet.[8]

When he had invoked the Greeks on the subject of feet, Dr Zacharie had not been obliged to look back over the years to the teaching of Dr Andrew Combe, for doctors no less than artists had found in Greek art a continuing source of inspira-tion. In 1880, for instance, Dr George Wilson of Edinburgh had published his *Healthy Life and Healthy Dwellings* (subtitled, A Guide to Personal and Domestic Hygiene) and in discussing exercise for women had directed those in charge of growing girls to teach them

> not merely to understand the Greek tongue, but to copy somewhat of the Greek physical training, of the 'music and gymnastic' which helped to make the cleverest of the Old World the ablest race likewise ... they will then earn the gratitude of the patriot and the physiologist by doing their best to stay the downward tendencies of the physique, and therefore ultimately of the *morale*, in the coming generation of English women.[9]

Dr Wilson provided, furthermore, yet another reason for emulating the dress of the Greeks and the Romans:

> On physiological grounds, the classic mode was incomparably superior to the modern style of dress, because the whole weight of the garments was borne by the shoulders, and not from a waist constricted by strings and bands, if not by tight-laced stays. It may be true that the style of garments worn by Greek and Roman women may not be suited to our colder climate, but the closer the adaptation of modern apparel is to that style, so much more artistic taste will be displayed, and the better will be the health enjoyed.[10]

In suggesting in his lecture held in the Health Exhibition of 1884 that Greek and Roman dress was beautiful but only practicable in England when worn over woollen combinations, E. W. Godwin was upholding views already fully expressed by members of the medical profession.

At the end of July a conference was held in the premises of the Healtheries designed to discuss conditions in schools, particularly in reference to over-work, but a number of doctors and others who were present took the opportunity of speaking on

other topics too. Reporting the conference, *The Times* referred
to Mr Treves who had, according to the *Lancet*, been the moving
spirit in the display of the scientific aspects of dress.

> Mr Treves' essay on dress will be instructive to many
> readers . . . in spite . . . of the formal assent which is generally
> given to any enumeration of the principles of wholesome
> dressing, it seems probably that the human race will require
> to be subjected to the influence of another century of civilisa-
> tion before they will universally, or even generally, repudiate
> the arrangements under which the fashionable forms of
> costume are now determined by a few highly placed per-
> sonages for the multitude; while they are determined, for the
> personages themselves, by the ingenuity of enterprising
> tradespeople who devise new combinations of attire with a
> single eye to the obtaining of enhanced profits in their
> business.[11]

One of the most important reforms urged by Godwin and all
those who spoke of hygienic dress was the wearing of wool next
to the skin, a practice long advocated by doctors who, even
before the middle of the 19th century, had insisted that flannel
should be worn as a part of the underclothing of both men and
women. The popularity of the red flannel petticoat had been a
result of this campaign. By the time the International Health
Exhibition presented its section on healthy dress, however, the
newer theories of Dr Jaeger were beginning to gain ground and
natural wool, unbleached, and knitted (by hand or machine),
worn next to the skin, was replacing flannel. Essays and lectures
on his 'System', translated from the German of Dr Jaeger had
reached England from Stuttgart before the Health Exhibition
was planned, and the type of garment he advised was, itself,
shown in the Exhibition. In 1887 a revised and greatly enlarged edition, with the title *Essays on Health Culture*, was
published in London by Waterlow & Co, who had been
responsible for printing all the publications for the Health
Exhibition.

The power of Dr Jaeger's arguments was greatly enhanced by

the fact that he began by declaring frankly that he had tried them out on himself and had been transformed thereby from a sick man to one who was relatively healthy. As a result of a leg-injury, leading to blood-poisoning before he was thirty, his enforced sedentary life had meant that

I gradually grew fat and scant of breath; my digestion was disturbed; I suffered from haemorrhoids, and was troubled by a tendency to chill diseases.[12]

Since, in this state of health, he was appointed to lecture to the Stuttgart Royal Polytechnic on anthropology and zoology, Dr Jaeger felt that, as a physician, he ought to heal himself first. Short essays on his progress towards recovery had appeared, reprinted chronologically in earlier works so that, in consequence, he was able to claim in his foreword to his enlarged and revised edition that

the experience of many thousands of wool wearers in every country and climate under the sun has added new and valuable information as to the hygienic worth of my System, which has the happy faculty of attracting the enthusiastic interest – I had almost said affection – of those who adopt it.[13]

The importance of disposing of poisons in the body through the exhalations of the skin and the equal importance of getting rid of flabby fat, were both thoroughly understood by 19th-century doctors, many of whom, especially Germans, had put forward various ways of doing so. Dr Jaeger lists some of them including, for instance, 'healing gymnastics' (impossible for those too weak to undertake them) and Turkish baths (not always available and when they were, only to the rich). The treatment advocated by Dr Banting, the subject of an exhibit in the Healtheries, Dr Jaeger also disapproved of, saying that the attempt to cure the evil of surplus adipose tissue by the avoidance of certain foods could be dangerous, 'whereas by maintaining and assisting the activity of the skin the water is drained from the body, reducing or thickening the mass of bodily juices'.[14]

Dr Jaeger, who was manifestly fond of his food, not only advocated the wearing of wool next to the skin for the purpose of encouraging perspiration, but he regarded the wearing of vegetable fibres and of silk, too, as positively injurious to health, and explained his reasons for this view. No animals other than man, he pointed out, wore linen or cotton for their covering and silk was, after all, not a natural covering but the excretion of a worm. Living vegetables collected the excreta of animals and transformed them into matter healthy to man. Dead vegetable fibres, on the contrary, absorbed noxious vapours when cold and gave them off, equally noxious, when conditions became warm, thus poisoning the air. Wool, hair, and feathers behaved very differently. They absorbed noxious exhalations and transformed them into wholesome sweetness.

Straightforward as Dr Jaeger's theories were and correct as they may have been, they made great demands on his faithful 'Woolleners', for not only to restore health to the sick, but once cured to keep them healthy, meant that absolutely nothing that was not an animal product could be worn, and even those must be treated in special ways. All garments worn over the basic woollen covering (of shirt and pants or the combinations in which the two were joined into one garment) must also be made entirely of wool, since even a partial cotton lining would inevitably prevent some of the bodily exhalations from escaping, and drive them back upon themselves.

In his *Health Culture* published in English in 1887 – which, he said, he was writing in 1885 – Dr Jaeger dealt separately with each garment in the masculine and feminine wardrobes. Some of his theories on men's dress will be discussed in chapter 8, but, speaking generally, what he had to say about the basic clothing of one sex applied to the other also. With German thoroughness he omitted nothing and was just as precise in describing healthy hats as other more intimate articles of clothing. Of women's hats [36] he says:

the materials employed should consist only of woollen cloth,

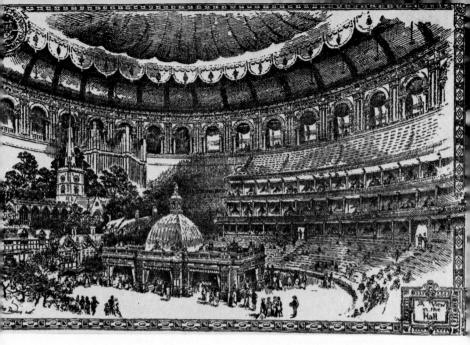

32. International Health Exhibition, 1884. Inside the Albert Hall; historical and Rational dress was exhibited round the galleries. From the souvenir to the Shakespeare Show.

33. An artist's impression, emphasising the international aspect of a soirée at the Health Exhibition. *Graphic* 1884

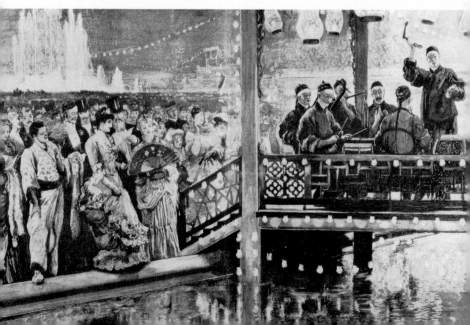

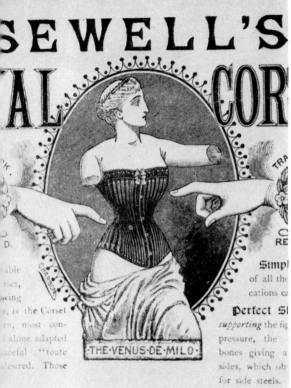

SEWELL'S
AL COR
THE·VENUS·DE·MILO

34. Advertisement for the Survival Corset in the souvenir of the Shakespeare Show at the International Health Exhibition in 1884

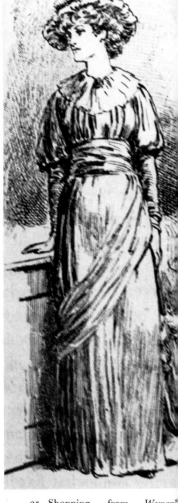

35. Shopping, from *Woman's World*, 1888. A young lady wearing an artistic dress chooses a Liberty silk. Compare her dress with that worn by Mrs Michael Chapman, figure 58

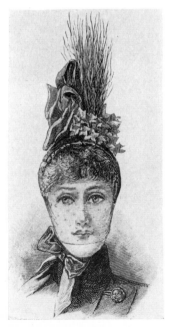

36. Black horsehair bonnet, from *Woman's World*, 1888. A flattering but fragile bonnet composed of natural materials.

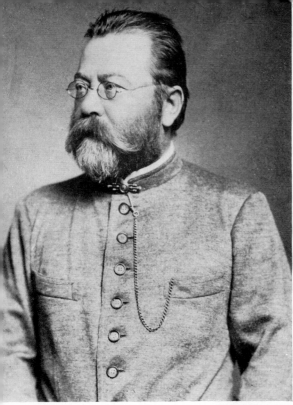

37. Dr Gustave Jaeger wearing a sanitary woollen suit

38. Two versions of Dr Jaeger's digital socks

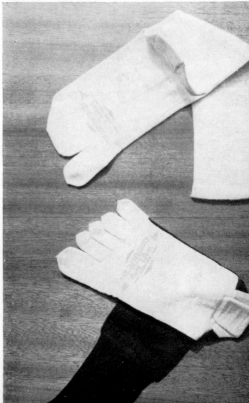

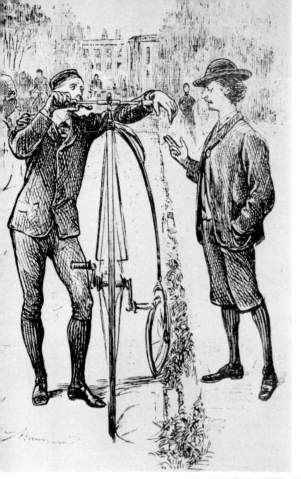

39. The Line of Beauty. George du Maurier. *Punch* 1879. Knee breeches, a fashion shared by athletes and aesthetes.
Athlete: 'Don't you bicycle?'
Aesthete: 'Er – no. It develops the calves of the legs so! Makes 'em stick out you know! So coarse! Positive deformity'

40. Sic Transit. George du Maurier. *Punch* 1893. Knee breeches as a mark of the progressive intellectual. 'By the way, Duchess, supposing that we *do* succeed in getting the House of Lords abolished this season, won't it be a great blow to the Duke?' 'Yes, if he ever hears of it; but I shan't tell him, you know!'

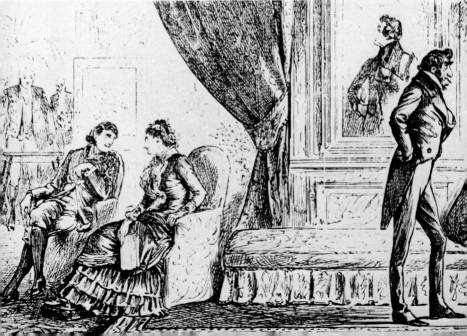

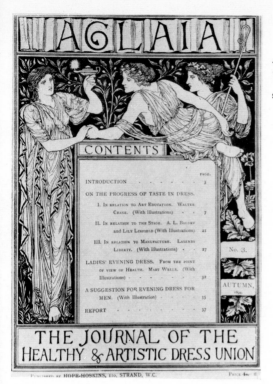

41. Cover design by Henry Holiday for *Aglaia*, no. 3, Autumn 1894. The first number, with the same cover, appeared in July 1893

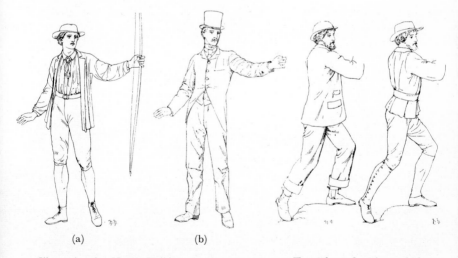

(a) (b)

42. Illustration by Henry Holiday. In the pose of Apollo Belvedere, a man (a) in ideally comfortable and aesthetically pleasing clothing is compared with (b) the typical costume of the 1890s, suitable only to 'money-making machines'. *Aglaia*, Spring 1894

43. Towards a reform in men's dress; (right) another suggestion designed by Henry Holiday. *Aglaia*, Spring 1894

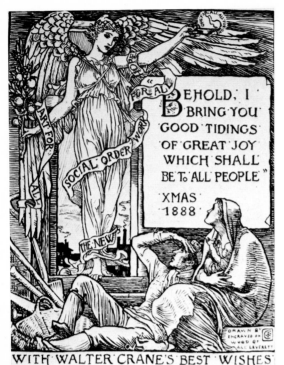

44. Walter Crane's design for his own Christmas card for the year 1888 in which he calls not only for 'work for all' but also for 'art for all'. This was the year in which *Robert Elsmere* was published

45. Art in Whitechapel. Loan Exhibition of Pictures in St Jude's School House, Commercial Street. *Graphic*, November 1884. This was obviously the inspiration for the scene in *Robert Elsmere*. (See appendix 2)

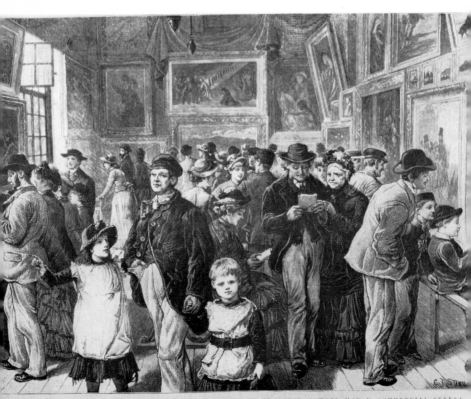

ART IN WHITECHAPEL—LOAN EXHIBITION OF PICTURES IN ST. JUDE'S SCHOOL HOUSE, COMMERCIAL STREET.

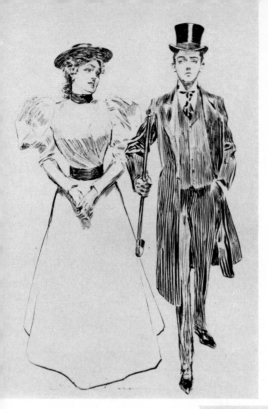

46. 'Who is the best dressed man in your college?'
'Well Tom Goldage is the *second* best.' The return to conventional dress at the end of the '90s. Charles Dana Gibson. *Drawings 1898*. (See figure 49)

47. This Can Happen, detail. Charles Dana Gibson, 1898. Pretty, conventional well-to-do American girl wearing a dress inspired by masculine fashions. *Drawings 1898*

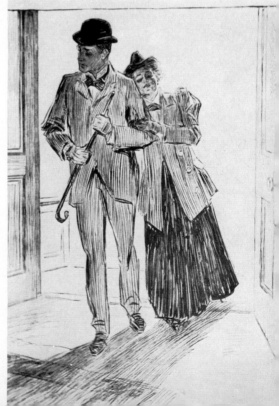

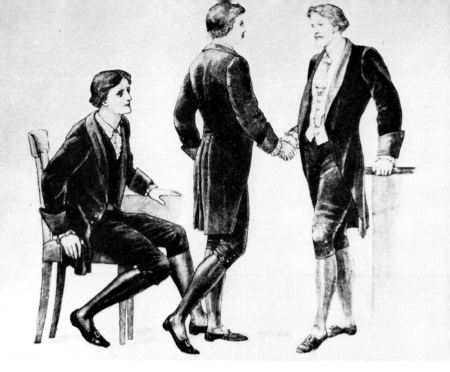

48. Improved evening dress for Gentlemen, a step towards better taste. *Aglaia* 1894

49 Counter-reformation; male intellectual of the '90s returns to conventional dress clothes. George du Maurier. *Punch* 1893

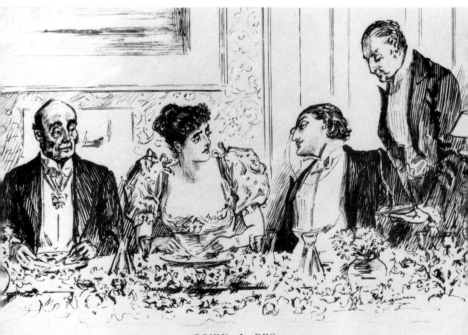

DOWN A PEG.

Mr. Gifted Hopkins (Minor Poet, Essayist, Critic, Golfer, Fin-de-Siècle Idol, &c.) "OH, MRS. SMART—A—I'VE BEEN THINKING, FOR THE LAST TWE
NUTES, OF SOMETHING TO SAY TO YOU!"
Mrs. Smart (cheerfully). "PLEASE GO ON THINKING, MR. HOPKINS,—AND I'LL GO ON TALKING TO PROFESSOR BRAYNE IN THE MEANTIME!"

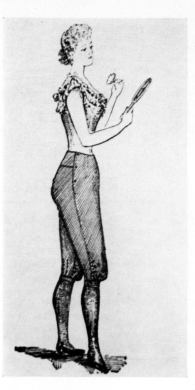

50. Capper's Csandco Hygienic Knickers. Advertisement in *Aglaia* Autumn 1894. 'This Artistic and Hygienic Garment is scientifically cut . . .'

51. The Athenian gown. Advertisement in *Aglaia*, Autumn 1894. Described as a classical Greek tea-gown in soft French crêpons

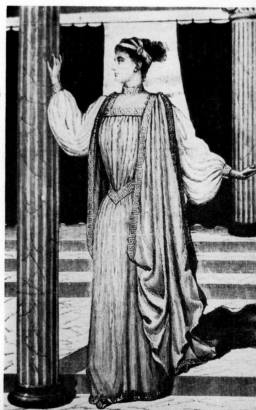

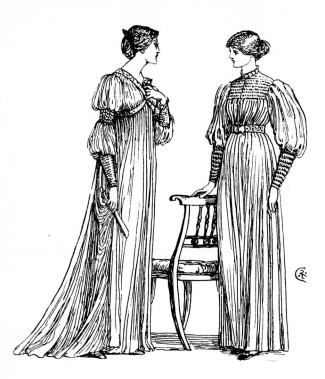

52. Types of Artistic Dress. Walter Crane. *Aglaia* 1894. Two dresses closely resembling these were advertised in Liberty's catalogue several years later

53. 'Trilby'. George du Maurier. Published 1895. Wearing Grecian dress, Trilby sings Ben Bolt on the stage of Drury Lane Theatre

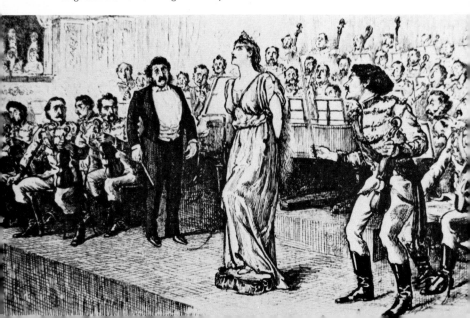

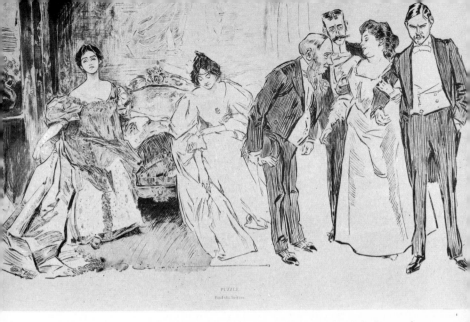

54. Puzzle: Find the Heiress. Fashionable American girls wearing artistic dress and hair-dressing. Charles Dana Gibson. *Drawings 1898*

55. Rational Costume. George du Maurier. *Punch 1896*. Young girls of the upper-class wearing masculine bicycling dress in the '90s. Vicar: 'It is customary for men, I will not say *Gentlemen*, to remove their hats on entering a church'

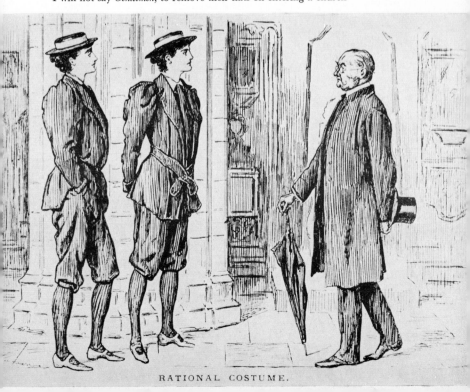

RATIONAL COSTUME.

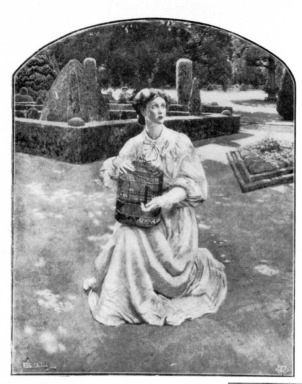

56. 'Caged Bird', 1907. Byam
Shaw. An allegory; the bird is
freed by the 'caged' woman
who wears a dress influenced
by earlier PreRaphaelite
designs

57. 'L'Education sentimentale'. Aubrey
Beardsley. The Yellow Book Vol. I. The
young girl wears the high-waisted artistic
dress of the 1890s

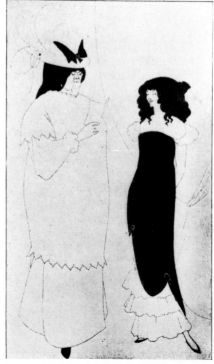

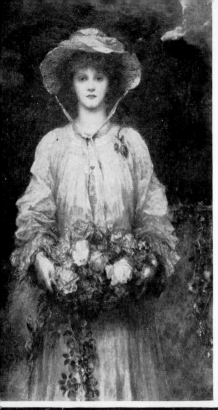

58. 'Lilian' (Mrs Michael Chapman) by G. F. Watts. The Watts Gallery. Soft draped artistic dress worn at the end of the '80s

59. 'A Woman's Protest'. Byam Shaw. Inspired by a poem by Arthur Hugh Clough posthumously titled 'A Protest'. (See appendix 1)

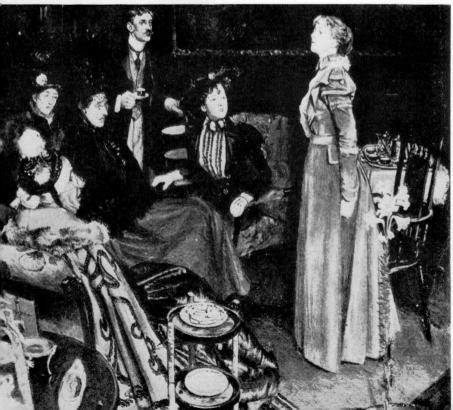

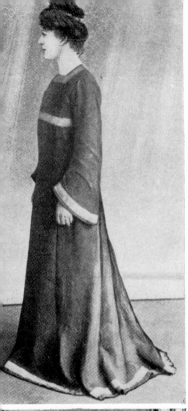

60. In contrast to van der Velde's design (figure 62), this German dress of 1903, although probably worn by an upper-class woman is, nevertheless, more democratic in intention. From *Frauenreform Kleidung*

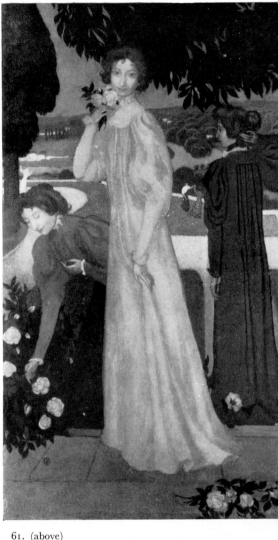

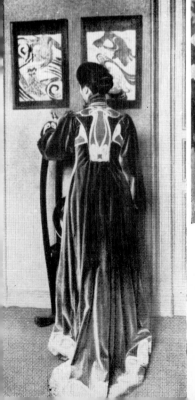

61. (above)
'Mademoiselle Yvonne Lerolle' in three poses, 1897. Maurice Denis. In the centre and on the right she wears artistic dress. Daughter of the painter, Henri Lerolle, the sitter belonged to the French artistic set

62. (left) Projet de robe, about 1896. Henry van der Velde. A luxurious 'artistic' dress designed by a well-known Belgian artist

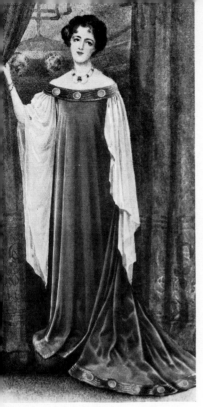

63. Iseult. *Liberty catalogue*, 1905. Evening gown of supposedly 'mediaeval' inspiration

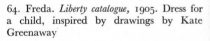

64. Freda. *Liberty catalogue*, 1905. Dress for a child, inspired by drawings by Kate Greenaway

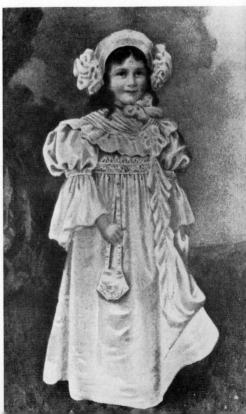

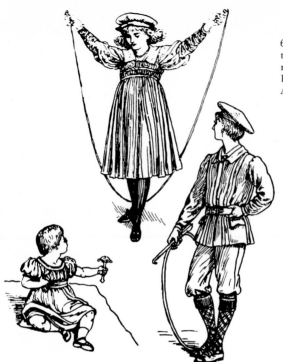

65. 'Utility, simplicity, picturesqueness'; types of children's dress designed and drawn by Walter Crane. *Aglaia*, Autumn 1894

66. Cover for souvenir programme of the May Day processions, 1907, urging adult suffrage by Walter Crane. Crane shows Liberty as a working-class girl wearing an apron and almost identical dress to the girl's on the cover for *The Woman Worker* which first appeared in 1907 and was also designed by him

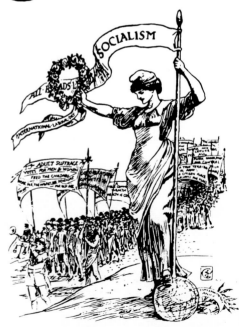

A SOUVENIR FOR MAY DAY 1907

or felt, or horsehair. With these materials, and with feathers, and ornaments derived from the animal and mineral kingdom, hats may be made which are both hygienically and aesthetically irreproachable, while avoiding unsanitary materials, and injurious, poisonous dyes.[15]

Women's collars and cuffs he found no fault with, providing they were made of wool, cashmere, or woollen lace, nor did he disapprove of occasionally wearing a low-cut neckline, since the neck is not particularly sensitive and is much more hardened to resist the effects of exposure than it would be if the wearer were not sanitarily clad:

> It should, however, be a strict rule that the neck of the dress should be equally low behind as in front, so that the proper distribution of the blood suffer no interruption, as it must do if the dress be cut low only in front.[16]

The licence to wear low-cut necklines is surprising since Dr Jaeger very much disapproved of draughts. He liked long, tight-fitting sleeves; but if short sleeves were worn then long woollen or undyed leather gloves should be worn with them, and men would do well to draw their gloves over their coat-sleeves so that any draught might be excluded. He did not disapprove of the corset, a means, as he called it, of 'Girding the Loins'. This practice, he insisted, was hygienically correct for the fault did not lie in the corset, as so many had thought, but in the fact that it was made of the wrong stuff, that is to say, of vegetable fibre. Ladies who wore the Sanitary Woollen Corset, 'need use no force to preserve the shape; their compact firm figures will not require support'.[17]

Strict as he was, Dr Jaeger did not expect people to confine themselves always to dressing entirely in natural undyed wool: he allowed some colour. He pointed out, however, that since the wearing of wool next to the skin, which raises the temperature, activates further the poison emitted by noxious dyes, even greater care had to be taken by wool-wearers than by those who wore linen. Having invented what he named a system of 'nerve measurement', he was able to assess the damage done to each individual by the wearing of certain colours, for some colours affected some people adversely and not others.

> For summer clothing, working, and everyday costume, especially for any kind of athletic sport, as also in hot climates, the material should be entirely free from dye – i.e., natural white or natural brown . . . Dyed materials are least injurious in winter, in cold climates, when the body is in repose, and for Sunday visiting, and holiday attire (but not for dancing-exercise, which is a species of sport).[18]

Natural, vegetable dyes, so much loved by the aesthetes and, as we have seen, recommended in the section devoted to Dress in the Health Exhibition, were not approved of by Dr Jaeger. They faded, which was a great evil and, since the new aniline dyes faded too, they were equally condemned. Absolutely pure indigo and cochineal Dr Jaeger allowed, but they must be tested for purity, and any loose dye must be washed out. He freely admitted that it was difficult to get either an even weave or an even 'natural' colour in the woollen stockinet he recommended so highly: his System, he confessed, had met with great opposition from manufacturers. He bewailed the time when coats had been dyed with indigo only, and, though expensive, had been bought by peasants as an investment and bequeathed to their sons; it was impossible to produce pure woollen cloths of high quality cheaply and his adherents must be wary of buying cheap imitations. The goods he really approved of were made by his accredited manufacturers and bore a distinguishing trade-mark.

Health Culture includes a chapter on bathing: the Jews, Greeks, and Romans, who were Wool-wearers (a statement which might be questioned) bathed often, as Woolleners like to do; whereas those who wear linen have become so insensitive that they do not feel dirty and are satisfied with frequently washing their linen rather than themselves. Dr Jaeger also discussed, and to a great extent supported, vegetarianism which had become extremely popular in the 1880s among people with progressive views. The Health Exhibition had a vegetarian restaurant in its grounds and, although the reporter of the *Daily News* admitted that he had not ventured to try it, he had seen people who had done so coming away with smiles on their faces.

Dr Jaeger's shop in Regent Street, London, was, and still is, not far away from that which had been established in 1875 by Mr Lazenby Liberty, whose oriental textiles must, judging from the size and frequency of his advertisements in the *Queen*, have been a great success. Liberty sold Indian cashmeres and Madras muslins as well as silks of various thicknesses and weaves, many of them undyed but some dyed in a 'variety of rare artistic colours'. One of Liberty's advertisements, appearing in August 1878, had quoted the *Medical Examiner* as saying:

We can imagine nothing more delightful on a hot summer day than a complete outfit of oriental silk.[19]

In an advertisement that appeared in the following November the quotation was cut down to 'we can imagine nothing more delightful' as being, of course, more appropriate to the season.

Although Dr Jaeger claimed that his Woolleners were numerous and scattered widely round the world, there were certainly many people who supported the *Medical Examiner*'s opinion that nothing was more delightful than silk – to quote Dr Jaeger, 'only the excretion of a worm'.

Dr Jaeger's theory that the body should be closely protected from the air and sealed against draughts, was reflected, perhaps, in the exhibit mounted in the clothing section of the Healtheries by the Rational Dress Society under the presidency of the Viscountess Harberton, one of the supporters of the movement for women's enfranchisement. It was here that, besides evening and day dresses of a sensible but more or less orthodox kind, the notorious 'bifurcated garments' were to be found – divided skirts for both women and little girls. In 1884 it was not easy to persuade the public to take kindly to these; even the *Official Guide* was compelled to admit:

As a rule the innovators in ladies costume appeal more to the *reason* than to the *artistic* sense of those whom they seek to convert to their views, while at the same time they tax the courage and traditional prejudices of the fair sex to an extent that will probably place insuperable difficulties in the way of their efforts. Possibly if the artistic side of the question were kept more in view the difficulties now experienced by dress reformers would to a great extent vanish.[20]

The same objection was raised to hygienic boots and shoes which were a separate exhibit:

Boots and shoes occupy a considerable section in the Quadrant; unfortunately, however, the more hygienic the reputed qualities of the boot the less does its form commend itself to artistic taste.[21]

The *Official Guide* to the International Health Exhibition was under no obligation, of course, to define 'artistic taste' but it would have been nice if it could have brought itself to do so.

The Rational Dress Society had been formed in 1881 as the result of a meeting between the Viscountess Harberton who had contributed an article published in the *Queen* recommending the divided skirt, and Mrs E. M. King whose sympathetic eye had been caught by Lady Harberton's recommendation. Mrs King had already given serious consideration to the subject of dress reform and had been invited to read a paper at the Health Congress held in 1881 in Brighton. Her paper, which had been called *Women's Dress in Relation to Health*, was expanded and published in 1882 as a paperback pamphlet at sixpence with the title *Rational Dress*, or the Dress of Women and Savages.

As its subtitle implied Mrs King, who quoted the newest theory that dress had its origins not in utility but in ornamentation, sometimes in the painful form of decorative gashes on the face, considered that it was time civilised beings gave up their addiction to disfiguring and hurtful ornament, although she did not despise other forms of personal adornment. Most of the issues she raised are no longer relevant, but both her arguments and her manner of presenting them are more attractive to the modern reader than is most of the literature on the subject by her contemporaries. Her descriptions of the bodily deformities produced by tight-lacing (based on doctors' case-books), which she called barbarous self-mutilation, carry conviction.

Mrs King regarded the chances of reforming the design of women's dress piecemeal as slight – a clean break with tradition, she thought, would have to be made. She quoted a Dr Richardson who had written in the *Gentleman's Magazine* in 1880:

> It is astonishing how resolutely the advanced professors of medicine . . . have denounced the practice of compressing the body in the stages of its growth . . . It is equally astonishing how resolutely the votaries of fashion have resisted the teaching of the learned.

On the other hand, thought Mrs King:

> The sensible-woman style of dress will never be adopted by young people. It is generally of no particular colour – and of no particular cut – it neither follows nature nor art . . . what is the use of the sensible elderly woman clothing herself in a healthy dowdy manner except in so far as her own comfort is concerned, if no young people can be induced to do like-wise?[23]

Men, Mrs King reminded her reader, had often declared that women seem to compensate for the necessity to hide the lower part of their bodies by the undue exposure of the upper part.

> Women always feel themselves in the position of being looked at rather than looking – the reverse is the case with men . . . Nothing will restore to women the proper equilibrium and healthy tone of mind . . . but a style of dress following equally and evenly the natural lines of the body, not suffering the half of it to be more hidden than the other, nor one part more displayed than the other . . . In proof of the truth of the theory that undue hiding of one part of the body leads to undue exposure and morbid desire for the display of the

other, let it be remembered that when tied-back skirts were in fashion, which allowed the outline of the lower limbs to be seen, waists were permitted to grow perceptibly bigger and low-necked dresses went very much out of fashion.[24]

It may be remembered that Mrs Haweis, writing when these tied-back dresses were actually in fashion, though she had deplored the tying back (avoidable by good dressmakers), had regarded the dresses as both beautiful and comfortable since they followed the lines of the natural figure [16].

Mrs King admitted that it was no easy thing to start a system of dress reform

> founded on true ideas of beauty, for the taste of both men and women has been so long vitiated by the contemplation of bad models, that nearly all sense of what constitutes female beauty has been lost sight of ... the portraiture of the beautiful undraped form remains to be hung up on a wall, or elevated on a pedestal, a mark for the vulgar gaze of the many; but the form to be clothed is a thing we see in shop windows, in shape like an hour-glass.[25]

Mrs King's paper, when it was read to the Society of Social Science's Congress in Brighton the previous year, had evidently been very persuasive, for the Rational Dress Society, in its very earliest infancy when the Congress was held, was awarded the Society's silver medal.

In 1883, due no doubt to the combined efforts of Lady Harberton, who became its president, and Mrs E. M. King, who became its secretary, the Rational Dress Society, with several doctors on its committee, presented an exhibition of Rational Dress in the Princes Hall, Piccadilly. Its catalogue survives, illustrated by reproductions of a good many, though not, alas, all of the exhibits. Since it is almost certain that either these clothes or others very like them were shown in the section devoted to Rational Dress in the International Health Exhibition of 1884, it is from them that we can deduce the appearance of the bifurcated garments that proved so disturbing.

At this date, though not, as will be seen, five years later, it seems that 'bifurcated garment' was merely a euphemism for trousers or breeches worn beneath a skirt, but partly exposed. Sometimes, like the pantalettes that little girls had worn in the 'sixties, only a little of the trouser was allowed to show above the ankle, but at others the skirt reached only to about the knee and below it breeches extended to about half way down the calf, the rest of the leg being covered by stockings. Like all attempts to impose an artificially created fashion, few of the exhibits look any more attractive today than they did to most observers at the moment of their invention. The best of them are two 'dresses of the future', one rather like the masculine dress of the reign of Elizabeth I, the other a comic-opera version of an 18th-century man's dress with knee-breeches ending in lace frills. The exhibition at the Prince's Hall was divided into sectors in some of which commercial firms, such as Debenham and Freebody, were responsible for the display; Liberty's showed a collection of unloaded silks. Others were arranged by well-known dress-making establishments, some of them theatrical firms. Prizes were awarded by a number of panels of judges for various categories of dress. The main emphasis was on lightness – Grace & Cie, for instance, showed a dinner dress to be worn without stays which weighed no more than 3 lb 3 oz – but fitness for purpose was also taken into consideration. The house of M. E. Fisher, exhibiting boating, walking and tricycling dresses, added piquancy by including a 'Costume of "A Love Sick Maiden" (opera of "Patience")'.

An Edinburgh doctor, John Holm, apparently on his own initiative, showed a 'Calisthenic Dress' and the Head Master of a boy's school, also from Edinburgh, showed a shirt with a 'Loose Neck'. Eight 'Working Women's dresses' competed for a prize of £5 but the first prize of £50 was awarded to Madame Brownjohn who exhibited a 'Dress with Trousers', a theme which the organisers of the show were very anxious to press home.

The title-page of the catalogue to the Rational Dress Exhibition carried the Society's belief that, 'Clothing should follow and Drapery not contradict, the natural lines of the body'.[26]

Both the medical profession and those interested in other aspects of health must have considered the Piccadilly exhibition sufficiently impressive not only, as was announced in the preliminary speeches, to warrant the inclusion of a section on Dress Reform in the proposed International Health Exhibition to be held the following year, but also to entrust the organisation of it to the Rational Dress Society.

In 1885, a year after the opening of the Health Exhibition and certainly as a result of it, the *Science of Dress in Theory and Practice*, by Mrs Ada S. Ballin, was published. Mrs Ballin, like Mrs Haweis, tried to reconcile beauty and function but, fortified by the Health Exhibition, she was able to adopt a severer and more dictatorial tone. Mrs Ballin subscribed to at least some of Dr Jaeger's theories and found that wool was the natural clothing of man as well as of the lower animals and she stressed the danger of poisonous dyes, condemning, therefore, doctors who supported the idea that red flannel was desirable from the point of view of health (its colour was very much out of key with current taste but this Mrs Ballin did not mention). She followed Dr Jaeger in assessing the heat-value of colours and remarked that there was 'much to be said in favour' of toed-stockings. Naturally she also warned against the dangers of tight-lacing:

> We must have no garments fitting so tightly as to impede vital processes, none so heavy as to weary the wearer, none cut in such a way as to cramp her movements, and none dyed with poisonous substances. What we want is REFORM, not REVOLUTION.[27]

In Mrs Ballin's view current attempts at dress reform were failing because they directed their efforts towards those who were already so set in their ideas that conversion was impossible:

> The battle for dress reform is at the present time being very vigorously fought but the soldiers of the rebel camp have unfortunately adopted a mistaken plan of falling upon the enemy just where he, or rather she, is strongest.[28]

The only hope, she felt, was to start by educating children, and here she resorted to several quotations from Herbert Spencer on the subject of the education of the young. Mrs Ballin did not explain how, even if children were converted *en masse* to dress reform, they would be able to convert their parents to their point of view.

Two chapters of the *Science of Dress* were devoted to the new bifurcated garments, and here Mrs Ballin was distinctly more sympathetic and hopeful than the *Official Guide* to the Health Exhibition had been. She fell back on Dr Jaeger (who had never advocated the wearing of a divided dress for women, since he considered woollen 'drawers' quite adequate) in seeing that 'still greater advantage may be gained by clothing each leg separately, as the passage of cold air which takes place beneath petticoats is thereby avoided ... the principle of the divided skirt is by no means necessary'.[29]

She furthermore admitted that the *Lancet* had, in 1879, spoken in no uncertain terms on the subject of bifurcated garments: 'We consider this article of dress unnecessary, and in many ways detrimental to health and morals'.[30] That, after all, had been before the presentation of the Health Exhibition. Since then, Mrs Ballin was sure, divided skirts had become very much more popular. She even claimed, rather surprisingly, that they had in fact been gaining in popularity, though slowly, ever since the bloomer costume – a theory for which any substantial support seems very difficult to find. In her chapter headed Trouser Dresses, openly disagreeing with the opinion expressed in the *Official Guide*, Mrs Ballin claimed that 'A really elegant walking costume in cashmere and silk, with a divided skirt, was shown by Mrs Beck in the Healtheries, which hardly differed in appearance from ordinary dress'.[31] The assurance that this trouser-dress could hardly be distinguished from normal fashionable dress was surely an indication of the difficulty of launching this fashion.

The taste of those who clamoured for reform in women's dress and of those who opposed or were indifferent to it, can never have been so sharply divided as it was at the time of the opening of the Health Exhibition and the three or four years

that followed. The comparatively 'natural' composition of the
fashionable dress that had appeared in the late 'seventies and
could still be found as late as 1882 had completely disappeared
by 1884 when an uncompromisingly unnatural design replaced
it, one which, once again, could only be properly appreciated in profile. There was no return to the sweep of the
Grecian Bend provoked by the Watteau toilette; instead, in
profile, women now looked like hens with a small compact head
carried upright on a torso so closely fitted by its covering as to
appear almost armour-plated, and a square and apparently
solid projection below the waist at the back. If Monet had
caught the spirit of the 'sixties in his *Femmes au Jardin*, it was
Seurat in his *Grande Jatte* who most perfectly reported the dress
and the carriage that resulted from it in the middle 'eighties. [30]

In comparison with the Seurat fashion, the bunched and
drooping chignons and the cascades of frills and ribbons that
flowed over the crinolettes of the early 1870s look positively
romantic; and yet without the preparation provided by the
very remotely similar line of the early 'seventies, the hard and
precise shape of the orthodox dress of the middle and later
'eighties would appear even more extraordinary than it does. In
Frith's painting of the *Private View* [29] at the Royal Academy
of 1881 a more or less expert eye is necessary to distinguish
between those who do and those who do not wear artistic dress:
no such uncertainty could have been possible had he painted
the scene in 1885.

Wooden as the exteriors of these ladies of the 'eighties
appeared, all of them may have been Woolleners beneath. Dr
Jaeger must certainly have approved of their long tight sleeves
which allowed no draughts to ascend to the elbow, though
Watts may have found them sausage-like [31].

The split between Aesthetes and those who had come to be
called not only by Matthew Arnold but by any journalist,
Philistines, was popularly recognised but the barrier between
these two social groups was transcended by the change in
domestic life brought about by contemporary writers on
health and the arts, as well as by the Health Exhibition itself.
This was particularly true of interior decoration for, at about

this time, it can be seen that the look of the home itself had changed. Naturally, 'good' and 'bad' taste remained but both looked different.

Dr Jaeger had been as thorough-going in his condemnation of the use of vegetable fibres for bedding and all domestic furnishings as for clothes themselves: in this sphere his theories appear even more curious. Since he was convinced that vegetable-matter, unless alive, absorbed and gave off noxious vapours, he declared that it should either be completely banished from the home and place of work, or else sealed-off so that no evaporation could take place. Everything, therefore, must be made of wool, hair, leather or, since furniture itself required a harder substance, of metal. When wood was used it must be varnished, polished or painted, so that none of its natural surface might be exposed. No linen, cotton or silk should be tolerated. In theory this allowed the use of woollen carpets; but since the wool must be absolutely pure and associated with no vegetable-matter, carpets could not be woven on a linen or hemp warp, which excluded all but the most expensive imported oriental rugs. New floor-coverings, such as oil-cloth sealed by wax or varnish, or bare boards properly sealed all over their surfaces, were offered as a more practicable solution.

According to Dr Jaeger, therefore, all the lace-curtains, the chenille and velvet hangings and tablecloths, the silk-tasselled fringes, the *macramé* borders, the brocaded silks, must go; so must almost everything that was not natural in colour, for absolutely safe dyes were few.

Society, of course, no more followed Dr Jaeger in this than in its outer dress, but his influence cannot have been entirely negligible for his ideas coincided in many respects with those of other people who were concerned with hygiene. Carpets, heavy velvet hangings, tasselled fringes and *macramé* borders harboured dust and therefore germs – the prime enemies of those who advocated healthy living. Nor could they easily be cleaned for, on the whole, they were not washable. The followers of William Morris, as well as of the chemists who lectured at the Health Exhibition, though not afraid of vegetable fibres disapproved

entirely of poisonous dyes. Thus not only furnishings but many
wall-papers were condemned – the latter in favour of sanitary
distemper paint as a treatment for walls.

Although Dr Jaeger rejected all dyes which faded (most of
the recently invented aniline dyes were not fast and he also
distrusted almost all vegetable dyes) he did allow indigo, which,
though vegetable, was fast, and cochineal, which was animal,
but only in their purest forms and not mixed with logwood,
with which indigo was almost always blended. His natural
undyed wool was available only in creamy-white, camel and
other light browns, and the very dark brown of 'black' sheep
(which was not black), which meant that his colour-schemes
were necessarily very limited.

Arrived at by a different route, via, for example, Whistler,
whose influence would no more have been admitted by the
haute couture than Dr Jaeger's, these simple colour-schemes
coincided with the artistic taste of the time. William Morris
and his associates favoured vegetable dyes not because they
were vegetable but because the colours they produced were
muted and certainly less harsh than colours produced by aniline
dyes; and Morris himself seldom used violent contrasts of
colour, nor did he use many colours together.

The heavy 'mid-Victorian' draperies had disappeared from
fashion, too. Four-poster beds were disapproved of as insanitary
(they could harbour bugs) and the curtains which hung from
them excluded beneficial fresh air. By 1885 they had been
succeeded in almost every middle-class home belonging to the
younger generation by the hygienic iron or brass bedsteads
which had no fixtures for supporting curtains. At the windows
of such houses 'Venetian' blinds allowed for ventilation while
excluding light when necessary, and these, or oiled-linen
blinds, were approved of as being more hygienic than hanging
curtains. Carpets which covered the floor from wall to wall
were disapproved of since their edges, hard to reach with a
brush, were considered a possible breeding-place for germs,
whereas rugs, scattered on wooden parquet floors or oil-cloth,
were regarded as sanitary because they were easy to take up and
shake.

Taste in ornament changed too. The deeply incised carvings which usually decorated four-poster beds and other pieces of large furniture, including pelmet-boards, fashionable in the middle of the 19th century, were now regarded as dust-traps. The same was said of the heavily carved mock Elizabethan (or more usually, mock Jacobean) furniture, fashionable in the 'seventies, and the even heavier Teutonic pieces, reproductions of corresponding German periods which had been favoured in England in the same decade. The surfaces of the furniture of the 'eighties were flatter, their carved decorations confined to smaller areas and much less deeply cut. From engravings of rooms manifestly designed for the Philistine taste of the moment it can be seen that these incorporated as many of the changes as those rooms which were indisputably artistic.

The changes were invariably in the direction of simplicity which, from about this time, began to be regarded as a 'better' quality than complexity, a philosophy which has prevailed until today and is still cherished. Not that the rooms of the 'eighties were cleared of small and purely ornamental objects – far from it; but these too were different. Soft woolly mats, threaded with ribbons, no longer lay on every horizontal flat surface; their counterparts survived but were crocheted of cotton and were washable. Pendant fire-screens embroidered in wools disappeared, popular ornaments were harder in texture, made of bamboo, china or metal, and often imported from the East. It was especially in the choice of these that the owner's taste could be displayed: artistic taste preferred, for instance, collections of blue-and-white china – simple in colour scheme – to more random effects.

Finally, Nature itself was submitted to censorship. Dr Jaeger had already repudiated cotton and linen. Now what were described by a lecturer of the University Extension Board as 'vulgar vegetable forms' must be replaced, by discriminating people, by what he called 'simple field flowers'. The vegetable forms were a reference to the full-blown violently pink roses, bunched together with sky-blue convolvulus and purple gloxinias of the wall-papers and embroidered chair-seats of the 1850s. The simple field flowers were the honeysuckle and cornflowers of William Morris – who did not himself, however, scorn the peony and the complicated form of the columbine.

Against this background even the dress of high fashion became more comprehensible. It may have formed a bastion against reform and the reformers, its torso certainly resembled what Watts called a piece of pipe but it was as hard and precise as the terse commands of the reformers. Its surface was broken by no deep folds or elaborate mobile trimmings. If its wearers did not look exactly like simple field flowers, still less did they look like vulgar vegetable forms.

It is difficult to assess the influence of the European scene on the Paris *haute couture* from which conventional dress certainly drew its inspiration. The movement towards dress reform in France was negligible, but the importance of hygiene was recognised as acutely in the home of Pasteur as in England. Fashions in dress are never reluctant to assume a virtue though they have it not and although the high fashion of the middle of the 'eighties could never be described as hygienic it cannot be denied that its lines were clean.

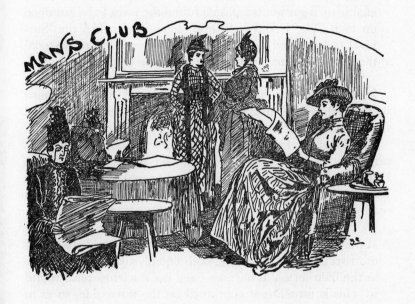

7

New Attitudes to Reform

The Rational Dress Society which had presented the controversial bifurcated garments at the International Health Exhibition in 1884, charged its members an annual subscription
of half a crown. In April 1888 the first number of its *Gazette*
appeared, at threepence, on page one of which it stated that the
maximum weight approved by the Society for underclothing
without shoes must not exceed seven pounds. It issued, furthermore, its own Rational System of underclothing which did not
follow Jaeger lines:

> Vest and drawers (or combinations) of wool, silk or the
> material called 'cellular cloth'. A bodice of some firm

material made high to the throat, to support the bust, and enable such garments as fasten round the waist to be buttoned on to it. The R.D.S's chemise (sometimes called the 'Survival'). A divided skirt made in whatever shape or material the individual may prefer; over this the ordinary dress.[1]

It will be noticed that no corset is included; it was replaced by the bodice of firm material to which drawers and divided skirt could be buttoned.

The first number of the *Gazette* also set out the Society's principles of dress, and included two articles, one on the Dangers of Women's Dress and the other on Why Women Age Rapidly as well as a paragraph on Divided Skirts which read:

It may be of convenience to our readers to be told that there are two makes of garments, both equally liked. That known as the 'Harberton' is narrow – and has a narrow pleat round it. This is usually not continued on the inner side, so as to avoid fulness between the ankles. The 'Wilson' is quite different. It is about a yard and a half round each leg. The pleats are carried up nearly to the waist, but so arranged as to fall outside the legs. Owing to the quantity of stuff required to make it, only very light materials should be used.
Patterns can be obtained at the Depot.[2]

The second type – the 'Wilson' – was named after Dr Wilson. Viscountess Harberton, who lent her name to the type first mentioned, was the president of the Rational Dress Society under whose auspices most of the exhibits that had dealt with reforms in dress shown at the Healtheries four years previously had been presented.

The Society's principles were such as one would expect:

The Rational Dress Society protests against the introduction of any fashion in dress that either deforms the figure, impedes the movement of the body, or in any way tends to injure health. It protests against the wearing of tightly-fitting corsets, of high-heeled or narrow-toed boots and shoes; of heavily weighted skirts, as rendering healthy exercise almost impossible; and of all tie-down cloaks or other garments impeding the movement of the arms.

It protests against crinolines or crinolettes of any kind as ugly and deforming.

The object of the R.D.S. is to promote the adoption, according to individual taste and convenience, of a style of dress based upon considerations of health, comfort, and beauty, and to deprecate constant changes of fashion that cannot be recommended on any of these grounds.[3]

The Rational Dress Society was anxious to deny the suggestion that it was out to persuade women to dress like men and it therefore continued to recommend the wearing of divided petticoats to those who did not wish to adopt divided skirts. Lady Harberton herself, however, while she did not wish women to look mannish always insisted that they should wear a bifurcated garment outside, either in the form of the 'Eastern Zouave' or the Japanese style of dress.

It may seem strange to us today that the aspect of Dr Jaeger's teaching which was taken most seriously was the importance of avoiding draughts up the legs rather than the wearing of wool which, since the *Gazette* repeatedly mentioned the new cotton cellular cloth, was apparently considered less important.

In 1888 all this seems very pedestrian and *dèja vu*. The extravagances of Dr Jaeger were disappearing; two patterns of the divided skirt could be bought, both designed to conceal its presence as far as possible. That was virtually all. The second number of the *Gazette* in which a meeting of the British Association was reported provides, however, a welcome little bomb. As a contribution to the discussion, Miss Lydia Becker, who had been a valiant participant in the battle for female emancipation in 1868 and was by this time aged 61, came out in favour of corsets. 'Stick to your stays', she had cried; 'they improve the form, give warmth and assist you. Stick to your stays, ladies, and triumph over the other sex'.[4]

The occasion had been the reading of papers on the Physio-logical Bearing of Waist-belts and Stays by two members of the Association. It is clear from the report in the Rational Dress Society's *Gazette* that Professor Roy and the surgeon, Mr Adaine, who presented the papers, had been expected to condemn the wearing of stays – doctors always had; but, in company with Miss Becker, they did not. An argument they put forward was at least original; it ran, according to the Gazette:

> They rather considered moderate tight-lacing as beneficial, as it released the blood from an *inactive* locality and left it free to be used in the brain and elsewhere.[5]

This new view was, of course, a direct reversal of the teaching of the revered Dr Andrew Combe, the famous Dr Beale and, more recently, of Dr George Wilson who in his dislike of corsets had gone so far as to advise some arrangement by which the whole weight of the clothing could be borne from the shoulders. This theory was expanded in a hand-book called *Dress, Health and Beauty* (manifestly of the middle of the 'eighties) in which a Shoulder-brace skirt and stocking supporter in one was advo-cated.

The recommendation of a laced corset by Professor Roy, Mr Adaine and Miss Becker had been strongly opposed at the meeting by Mrs Charlotte Stopes, a staunch supporter of dress reform, but the incident caused so much concern to members of the Rational Dress Society that Lady Harberton announced her intention of calling a drawing-room meeting for all members where the whole issue could be discussed.

In April 1889, the Rational Dress Society appealed for funds and also had pleasure in reporting that Mr Shimada, editor of the Tokyo *Daily News*, had sought the Society's help in bringing dress reform to Japanese women. In fact this was a political move which was defeated and had to be abandoned when the liberal government in Japan fell and its successor insisted that Japanese women should resume, or continue to wear, their national dress. Mr Shimada showed his appreciation of the

Society's work, however, by presenting it with the divided skirt of a Japanese gentleman in dark blue silk striped with black. The Society, as it happened, already had one made of cotton – it had been copied and launched as the 'Wilson'.

July 1889 seems to have seen the last number of the *Gazette* (it was replaced later by *Aglaia*, which will be discussed in succeeding chapters); its final issue included a long article which described the exotic, beautiful and comfortable clothing worn by Wagner and Balzac.

The Rational Dress Society's *Gazette* was a typical publication of a small and struggling association; it could not have been expected to survive. Far more impressive, indeed in quite a different category, was a new magazine launched in 1888, the same year as the *Gazette*, under the editorship of Oscar Wilde who was then in his early thirties. The title *Woman's World* was revived for this magazine, a tribute to the respect that must have been felt for the first *Woman's World* of the late 1860s. The twenty years that separated the two periodicals had not only brought a revolutionary change in the position of women but also in the quality of engravings, lithographs, and photogravures that could be used to illustrate publications of this kind.

There was nothing amateurish about the new *Woman's World* nor, clearly, any need for it to avoid articles on domestic topics; for women had by then become sufficiently sure of themselves to pursue, without apology, their own interests. The articles on cookery are good reading today, receipts at the same time simple and sophisticated show that the great mid-Victorian feasts were disappearing from the tables of intellectuals. Each number included two long illustrated articles on the current fashions in dress, the first on the London taste, the second on innovations in Paris. There were references to artistic dress but they were comparatively few and kept in perspective.

Since the names of contributors to *Woman's World* appeared not at the head of their articles but at the end, it comes as a recurring surprise when the names of women made famous by the parts they had played in the early days of the movement for

their enfranchisement, or in the struggles to attain equal professional standing with men, suddenly appear, following each
other as authors of successive intelligent articles; articles
which were by no means confined to domestic matters and the
majority of them still interesting today. Among the older names
are new ones: Ouida contributed several pieces, one on the
subject of war, and in later numbers the name of Marie
Corelli begins to appear. As well as writing editorials, notes,
and comments, Oscar Wilde regularly reviewed current
literature, especially poetry. He never handled with kid gloves
the women authors of whose books he disapproved.[6]

The two monthly features specifically devoted to the newest
fashions are interesting to the student of dress but there were
also occasional articles that discussed the clothes actually worn
by various types of women in society, and from these it can be
gathered that, in the later 'eighties, although both artistic and
rational dress continued to be worn by some women [58]
neither had increased in popularity. In November 1888 an
article appeared called Shopping in London. It recommended
a walk down Regent Street as a pleasant experience and, after
discussing various other kinds of customer, it devoted a long
paragraph to the type of girl to be found shopping at Liberty's
and reproduced a charming drawing of her [35]. Her looks are
based on the young Ellen Terry (who wore artistic dress herself), just as today the faces and postures of models in fashion
drawings and dummies in shop-windows are reminiscent of a
currently – or lately – popular star.

> Liberty's is the chosen resort of the artistic shopper. Note this
> lady robed in 'Liberty silk' of sad-coloured green, with rather
> more than a suspicion of yellow in ribbons, sash and hat
> (suggestive of a badly-made salad) who talks learnedly to her
> young friend – clothed in russet-brown, with salmon-pink
> reliefs showing in quaint slashings in unexpected places –
> of 'the value of tone', of negatives and positives, of delicious
> half-tones, and charming introductions of colour, fingering
> the while the art stuffs and *fade* silks shown her with a certain
> amount of reverence expressive of the artistic yearning of her

soul. We may be tolerably certain that such an one has her drawing-room arranged in the very last scheme of colour – cool silver-grey, possibly in conjunction with yellow terracotta and ivory, or the new red-brown with the faintest, palest of olive-greens ... Imagination further conjures up the lady herself in a tea-gown of silver-grey *pongee* cashmere, with full-front of yellow Surah; but when we find ourselves considering that terra-cotta and ivory silk would best suit her colouring and individuality, we mentally pull ourselves together, becoming aware that we are staring somewhat fixedly at the Artistic One. So we leave her deep in discussing with her friend and the Eastern-garmented shop-girl as to the relative merits of a sage-green or a dull red *portière* and pursue our character studies elsewhere.[7]

The *fade* background of the artistic drawing-room was considerably heightened by the addition of oriental rugs, Moorish-style furniture in dark wood, and huge Eastern pottery jars set in wrought-iron stands, all of which could also be bought at Liberty's.

In reality it was the eastern character of these artistic colour-schemes and not their *fade* tones which divided artistic taste from high fashion, for many fashionable clothes were *fade* too. An article of the same summer in the *Woman's World* described the latest bonnets in a tone from which, unlike the report on Liberty's, mockery was absent:

Natural materials are playing an all-important part in bonnets. The bright young face on this page is framed in one composed entirely of plaited pith ... it is of a pinky-string tinge ... So decidedly has Lady Fashion gone hand-in-hand with Dame Nature this year, that nothing in flowers is *à-la-mode* unless it looks as if it had just been gathered in the garden and tied up loosely, and there and then set in its place to stand erect, according to its own sweet will. Rushes from sedgy banks have been chemically treated and transferred to bonnets, with real grasses, real lavender, real rose-twigs. . . .[8]

Even in the *haute couture*, therefore, simple field flowers were preferred to vulgar vegetable forms.

Bonnets were of the greatest importance in the late 'eighties: fragile and vulnerable, they were the mark not only of the tastefully dressed but of the well-groomed woman. It is significant that in an article called *Dressing in Character*,[9] when the *Woman's World* described the clothes of the platform woman, it was her bonnet that gave her away. Because she might be called upon to address meetings in the morning, afternoon, and evening of the same day, the platform woman, according to the author, habitually wore black which was suitable for any occasion and, moreover, stood up to a good deal of wear and tear. At first glance she looked remarkably like any other lady, but when the eye caught sight of her bonnet she was betrayed.

In fact, simple and natural as their trimmings might appear, the bonnets of the late 1880s must have been the most appealing part of current fashionable dress though it is unlikely that their loosely knotted sprays of sedge-grass or their rose-twigs could humanise the characteristic exterior of the fashionable woman of the day. Compact and smooth as a hedgerow bird and as distinct in outline, she appeared, in her dress which gave no hint of soft flesh beneath, curiously utilitarian. The vulnerable nakedness was compressed into a mould that looked resistant, as the blackbird looks resistant. It was this woman, so severely condemned by dress reformers, rather than the melting artistic lady, who really proclaimed, with a cool precision, the victory of her sex. Wearing her pith-bonnet with its upright dagger of lavender that stabbed the air above her head, this woman combed her hair flat to her head and knotted it into a small tight relentless coil behind. Her tightly curled little fringe which hid the spring and growth of the hair on the forehead, so much admired by Watts, provided a perfunctory and strictly controlled decoration but no softness to her face. Beneath this severity, vapid faces look out from the fashion pages of the time; but it needs a second glance to see that they are, as they were designed to be, pretty. The only softness allowed to the fashionable woman of the later 'eighties was confined to this little oval area, so that it is not surprising that a 'hardening of the countenance' which speaking in public might produce, was to be feared.

In January 1889 the *Woman's World* published an article on Women Wearers of Men's Clothes, among whom Joan of Arc was, of course, the most famous. Speaking of contemporary French women, the author pointed out that although they had not emphasised the advantages of male clothing, when they did assume it they wore it with a more natural air than seemed possible in England. Breeches were commonly worn by Frenchwomen for *la chasse* (they had lately become very good shots), but the most prominent living Frenchwoman to take to masculine dress had been Madame Dieulafoy, who wore what the author described as a 'masher's suit' when she pursued her mission to Persian women in Shushan. Although at first the Shah of Persia had objected to receiving her in masculine dress, when her husband reminded him that she could never have carried out her work in any other costume he gave way and consented to meet her in her masher suit. Madame Dieulafoy had been working in appalling conditions, but 'No difficulty, no fever, no discouragement weakened her brave spirit'.[10] If, when she was wearing a masher's suit, Madame Dieulafoy met a lady, she felt it right to remove her hat.

What, however, asked Emily Crawford, the author of the article, had resulted from this wearing of men's dress?

Dr Mary Walker has talent enough to be anything in her profession, but she has not made a fortune in fees. Marie Dieulafoy's work was done in Persia and in a part of the country that has reverted to barbarism. Mrs Bloomer was clever, but what did her ability come to? Whereas Dr Elizabeth Blackwell, who was also clever and able, dressed like an ordinary sensible woman and was able to found a hospital.[11] [Headpiece to Chapter 7]

When the Rational Dress Society's *Gazette* disappeared, a demise which was not surprising if the view expressed in the article quoted was the popular one of the moment, *Woman's World* began to include paragraphs on the Society's work and various other activities among its editorial comments. By this time Oscar Wilde's name had disappeared from the cover and no other had taken its place. The tone of the reports on rational dress was not invariably sympathetic and on one occasion the editor went so far as to say: 'It cannot be denied that the opponents of dress reform find room for some little defence of the modern society woman's dress'. For, thought *Woman's World*, garments suspended from the shoulders as reformers recommended, endangered the collar-bone, and 'with a slight effort this little bone may be snapped'.[12]

An article by Mrs Charlotte Stopes was, however, allowed to adjust the balance, and when it appeared the editor offered to throw open the pages of *Woman's World* to a free discussion on the question of dress reform. Since no letters from correspondents appeared in subsequent numbers, nor any relevant articles, it seems that the subject was not, after all, as compelling as the editor had hoped. Meetings of the R.D.S. did, however, continue to be reported and it was soon possible to include the news, so satisfactory to reformers, that both Dr Lennox Browne and Dr Wilberforce Smith had declared that 'a wasp-like form, however desirable from the fashionable point of view can only be indulged in at the expense of the vital organs'.[12] This was followed, at the same meeting, by an attack by Lady Harberton on the drawings of Kate Greenaway, who, 'clothed the children of her fancy in "pretty" garments totally unsuited to the practical needs and comforts of boys and girls'[14].

If the cause of dress reform was not allowed to occupy much space in the *Woman's World* nor was the subject of women's enfranchisement. In 1884 the presentation of a new Bill in Parliament had shown that more than half the Members of the House of Commons were in favour of some form of women's suffrage. The Bill failed not for lack of support but because its supporters could not agree as to exactly which women should be enfranchised. Though to many women this must have been a bitter disappointment, it was less cruel than the earlier defeat of the 'sixties, for since then women had grown powerful enough to feel able to relinquish, at least temporarily, the fight for their enfranchisement in favour of other reforms that seemed even more urgent. Chief among these was what had come to be thought of as the scandal of class-discrimination.

Articles on this theme occupied a good deal of space in *Woman's World*. They included well-meaning but very mild pieces of advice to those hostesses who habitually gave parties to which they invited impartially their friends, their servants, and the local villagers. In these cases it was wise, the author thought, to ask a villager to act as joint host or hostess in order to put those who might be shy at their ease. She cited the case where a local cobbler (a 'time-honoured friend') had accepted this responsibility and prudently brought with him his collection of sea-weeds to engage the interest of people too timid to take part in the general conversation.[15] To the present generation it is difficult not to discern a tone of patronage in advice of this kind but it was off-set by the majority of articles which were far more weighty – those, for example, which suggested ways by which women of all social classes could earn a living. These included non-intellectual girls of the middle class for whom apprenticeships could be arranged with a guild of dressmakers set up for the purpose, which was to be run on the most business-like lines; 'we are strictly commercial and intend to "survive" on the Darwinian principle'.[16]

The suggestion that middle-class girls should become artisans is interesting; most authors were concerned to elevate, through education and opportunity, those of the working-class and especially to improve their working conditions and their wages, but it was class-distinction itself which began to be seen as a social evil at the end of the 'eighties. An article on 'Woman and Democracy', for instance, was, for its period, remarkably outspoken:

No elite subjects any more. . . . Woman has been the slave of man; and now she gives thanks for standing as spokesman of all the enslaved. The consciousness of belonging to a class is almost invariably lowering. . . . Class feeling is temporary, materialistic, external; it approaches so near to vulgarity, that any character which has a vulgar side shows that aspect when class interests are in question.[17]

Other writers, less philosophical in their approach, examined the relative advantages of time-work over piece-work in the employment of women – especially those who made shirts. One writer discovered that whereas every woman who went out to work, however poor, contrived to acquire a feather for her hat, it was by the condition of her boots that her standard of living could be judged. A glance at the boots of the women employees in a work-room could show whether their wages were adequate or not. Types of employer were carefully scrutinised, and while a few could be found who treated their employees well, the majority certainly did not.

For most of the social evils, education was regarded as the cure. By the end of the 'eighties, attempts to make higher education available to everybody outside the Universities included country-wide University Extension Lectures for which the charges were extremely moderate. Already, by this time, 'settlements' had begun to be established in working-class districts which could provide physical space where people could meet together to talk and to listen to talks. Immediately after Arnold Toynbee's death in 1883, a group of his friends and associates had opened Toynbee Hall in the Commercial Road, and in 1889 Mrs Humphrey Ward, with the co-operation of the Countess Russell and Mrs Frances Power Cobb, an early supporter of Women's Rights, had been the instigator of a University Settlement in Gordon Square on the lines of Toynbee Hall. The event was noticed by *Woman's World*, which described Mrs Ward's 'new Toynbee Hall . . . to be a centre for a school of thought rather than any given religious body'.[18]

Mary Augusta Ward had gained considerable fame in 1888, the previous year, from the publication of her three-volume novel, *Robert Elsmere*, the subject of a long and admiring analysis by Mr Gladstone in the *Nineteenth Century*. *Robert Elsmere* was not only a great success but was indisputably the book of the day – both serious and topical. Education, class discrimination, the current attitudes to the prevailing shades of English Christianity, the position of women, and even artistic dress are all dealt with in a convincing way. Its main plot investigates the struggles (particularly with his conscience and his noble-minded wife, Catherine) of a young clergyman who gives up a living in the Church of England to work among the ignorant poor in south-east London. His enthusiasm and his attractive personality draw round him a group of wealthy people as well as a cynical bachelor friend – Elsmere's former tutor at Oxford – who help him towards the foundation of just such a quasi-religious Settlement as Mrs Ward herself brought into being a year later. The issue was a perfect example of the current controversy on Faith versus Works, one of the most deeply discussed problems of the day.

The sub-plot was equally topical for it showed the determination of Catherine Elsmere's young and delicious sister, Rose, to establish herself as a top-rank professional violinist. She represents the ideal girl of the end of the 'eighties. Robert Elsmere's conscience is further tormented by this situation for, in his fanatical determination to draw all well-meaning people into the battle against poverty and ignorance, he sees even the arts as unnecessary luxuries.

Rose Leyburn makes her appearance very early in the book, before Robert's marriage to her saintly elder sister, Catherine. The three sisters (for there is a third, Agnes) share their Westmorland home with their mother. When the 'flourishes and broad *cantabile* passages' of one of Spohr's *Andanti* had ceased, 'a slim creature garbed in aesthetic blue, a mass of reddish brown hair flying from her face' stepped out into the garden to join Agnes, who remarks: 'And as for you Miss Artistic, I should like to know what you've been doing for the good of your kind since dinner'.

Agnes is described as wearing a dress which 'bespoke a young woman who respected both herself and the fashion'; whereas Rose was 'guiltless of the smallest trace of fashion. Her skirts were cut with the most engaging naïvete, she was much adorned with amber beads and her red brown hair had been tortured and frizzled to look as much like an aureole as possible. But, on the other hand, she was a beauty, though at present you felt her a beauty in disguise.' Rose replied to Agnes by throwing herself on the grass where she 'began to fling the fir cones lying about her at a distant mark with an energy worthy of her physical perfections and the aesthetic freedom of her attire'.[19]

In this early phase in her life Rose speaks of herself as wearing 'aesthetic' dresses. After Catherine's marriage she contrives to get some musical tuition in Manchester and later she pleads successfully for permission to go to Berlin. On her way there she visits the Elsmeres in their Surrey parish. The

> Rose of Long Whinsdale had undergone much transforma-
> tion. The puffed sleeves, the aesthetic skirts, the naïve
> adornments of bead and shell, the formless hat which she
> pleased to imagine "after Gainsborough" had all dis-
> appeared. She was clad in some soft fawn-coloured garment
> cut very much in the fashion, her hair was closely rolled and
> twisted about her lightly-balanced head; everything about
> her was neat and fresh and tight-fitting. A year ago she had
> been a damsel from the "Earthly Paradise"; now, so far as an
> English girl can achieve it, she might have been a model for
> Tissot.[20]

No description could better express the two points of view of the time. With her puffed-sleeves and her frizzled aureole of red-brown hair, Rose had worn exactly what Mrs Haweis had established as PreRaphaelite dress and what, it is fascinating to discover, had remained almost unchanged for more than a decade. In her transformation she wears the 'fawn-colour' so like the 'pinky-string' of the pith bonnet described in the *Woman's World* and everything about her was not only neat but tight fitting.

Back from Berlin, with a brilliant musical future before her, though poised and exquisitely stylish, Rose had lost nothing of her eager vivacity. If she, however, had abandoned her artistic pose, aesthetic dress does not disappear from the novel for it is still affected by Mrs Pierson, a climbing London hostess. She 'was small, untidy, and in all matters of religious or political opinion "Emancipated" to an extreme'.[21] She gives a party in honour of Rose at which among those present are a poet, a 'cellist 'with the hair', a lady in Greek dress, and an esoteric

Buddhist. Catherine Elsmere, acting as chaperone to her sister, writes to Robert about the gathering:

> As to Mrs Pierson, I never saw such an odd bundle of ribbons and rags and queer embroideries as she looked . . . However, Rose says that, 'for an aesthete' – she despises them now herself – Mrs Pierson has wonderful taste, and that her wall-papers and her gowns, if only I understood them, are not the least like those of aesthetic persons, but very *recherché* – which may be.[22]

Together with Emily Crawford's view that women could function more successfully dressed as 'ordinary women' than in reformed dress, Lydia Becker's 'Stick to your stays', and the *Woman's World's* patronising attitude to women who shopped at Liberty's, Rose Leyburn's later rejection of her teen-age craze for aestheticism is significant. It is doubtful whether, in 1889, Watts would still have been asked to write seriously on 'Taste in Dress' for a journal such as the *Nineteenth Century*, by which time many of the ideas put forward for a reform in the design and construction of women's clothes were in the course of being quietly and unobtrusively absorbed into the normal wardrobe. Others would be adopted before long and those that remained, although they continued to be affected by some enthusiastic young maidens with artistic leanings and by some women who wished to make themselves conspic-uous by striking progressive attitudes, were still in danger, or perhaps in renewed danger, of being treated with Gilbertian disrespect.

The new spirit that had found so acute an analyst in Mrs Humphrey Ward had its new types of heroes and heroines. For instance, although little more than twenty, Rose had come back from Berlin, whither she had been allowed to go on her own, utterly changed:

> What a personage she had grown in these twelve months – how formidably, consciously brilliant in look and dress and manner.[23]

Used of a girl of the late 'eighties, 'formidable' could be a compliment. The word could not have been applied to *Lothair's* heroic and active Mrs Campian (fearsome as she was) in 1870, and, earlier still, judging from the intellectual dialogues of the first *Woman's World* of the late 1860s, it had been essential to include a middle-aged Aunt to express in words sentiments that could be regarded, even distantly, as formidable. Young girls in the crinoline's dying fall could certainly not have been allowed to be 'consciously brilliant'.

In 1888, the hard sheath of the fashionable creation put out by the *haute couture*, with its fiercely sprouting crinolette, so 'formidable' in silhouette was, nevertheless, beginning to undergo a transmutation. In Paris what was named a 'Directoire' style was replacing it which, in its earliest stages, seems to those who look back today to represent hardly any change at all; but the very fact that it had been given a label from the past is an indication that the new fashion was thought of as more picturesque than its predecessor and it did, indeed, soften itself sufficiently to include large hats rather like those of Gainsborough's last sitters, and floppy frills about the neck and bosom.

It was probably no accident that Rose Leyburn, in her aesthetic period, had worn a hat that she regarded as based on Gainsborough's works; for the study of dress reveals that, as in all the arts, motifs, phrases, and sometimes even whole compositional ideas are in due course snatched by popularisers and pasticheurs and reissued in terms acceptable as the latest thing. It was only a matter of a few years before the naturalism of William Morris's decorative vegetation was mounted as the rushy sedges and hedgerow grasses of fashionable bonnets, and that aniline dyes were discarded in favour of quiet harmonies composed of mutations of the same 'impure' colour.

As for Robert Elsmere himself he, too, was the new hero – the post-Health-Exhibition parson: '"I will make myself a public nuisance, but the people shall have their drains",' said Robert to Langham, his old tutor and friend. '"It seems to me", said Langham musing, "that in my youth people talked about

Ruskin; now they talk about drains". "And quite right too. Dirt and drains . . . It's all very well, but they are the foundations of a sound religion". "Dirt, drains and Darwin", said Langham, meditatively, taking up Darwin's *Earthworms*, which lay on the study table beside him, side by side with a volume of Grant Allen's Sketches."[24]

In his work among the poor, Elsmere's chief supporter was the Hon. Hugo Flaxman, nephew of a duke, a younger son but immensely rich in his own right. Before winning a mathematics prize in Berlin he was known at Cambridge as 'Citizen Flaxman' from his habit of dining his scout or, when at home, dining with his servants and of shaking the hands of his friends' butlers. He is typical of one kind of support on which, in its early days, the English Socialist movement relied. Now, with the help of an aunt, he was collecting paintings from the various seats of his family for an exhibition in the East End and giving readings from the classics to Elsmere's gatherings of working-men [45]. Class snobbery was out – it was the target for half the jokes in *Punch* for the year 1888, which usually took the form of snobbish remarks dropped between dances from the lips of vapid young men in immaculate tails to beautiful but unsympathetic girls.

In this world that ended the earnest 'eighties, Philistine and Aesthete still jostled each other, intermarrying and begetting children of mixed beliefs and tastes. Most members of the upper and middle-class who were concerned with social reform, unlike Robert Elsmere, encouraged the arts since, putting them at their lowest, they were seen to have an educative and elevating effect on members of the working-class, so deserving of the best in life [44]. Nevertheless at the same time that the richest music and the most exalted literature were placed before the poor – nothing could be too good – in material things those which were humble seemed, somehow, better than those which were gorgeous. Thus wool 'art' serge was more admirable than Lyons velvet and hand-thrown earthenware superior to Sèvres china in the eyes of those with social consciences or artistic taste.

Social consciences were sprinkled widely through the literature of the moment. In the year 1888 which saw the publication of *Robert Elsmere*, a quite different kind of book came out by an Americano-English authoress, Mrs F. Hodgson Burnet. *Little Lord Fauntleroy* was no less successful than *Robert Elsmere*; it was praised by *Punch* for being good but without goody-goodiness and cant – it was, according to *Punch*, sincere. Its hero, a little boy born in the United States of an English father, son of an Earl, and an American mother, was described as dressed in a suit that very closely resembled that worn by Oscar Wilde on his American lecture tour six years earlier, though this the author seems not to have realised. The book's illustrator was highly sensitive to the latest artistic movements: for instance, the old Earl was shown seated in his castle rather implausibly in front of a Japanese screen, and in at least one of the rooms of this stately residence a strange writhing object like an embryonic specimen of the hardly yet formulated *art nouveau* appeared among the furnishings.

Fauntleroy, admittedly, was not dressed in art serge, but in other respects he was a child of his time. His favourite friends in America had been a boot-black and a small-shop grocer, with whom he kept in touch after coming to England; and as soon as he was in a position to impress his sentiments on the hitherto embittered Earl, his grandfather, he persuaded him not only to re-house such tenants as were living in bad conditions but also to give a huge party for all the tenantry at which the little boy made a speech of welcome. If this is not altogether today's version of democracy, the fact that in such a book as *Little Lord Fauntleroy* it forms an important part of the plot is an indication that the theme was popular. It was an aspect of the book which was soon recognised, for in 1895 *Punch* published a drawing of an apocryphal incident in the life of a little Lord, identical in appearance to Fauntleroy who, standing on a river bank, implores his governess to let him join a crowd of rowdy, uncouth and unappetising urchins precariously stuffed into a small boat.[25]

Like Rose Leyburn, *Punch* in 1888 had lost interest in ladies wearing healthy or artistic dress, which was unfortunate in the year of the inauguration of the Rational Dress Society's *Gazette* – mockery is better than total neglect; *Punch* was behaving like a spiteful woman in Mrs Humphrey Ward's novel, who remarked of a rival:

> She is East Ending. We all do it nowadays. It is like Dizzy's young man who "liked bad wine, he was so bored with good".[26]

If, at the end of the 'eighties, female dress reform had ceased to be a topical issue, comfortable, healthy and childlike dress for little boys and girls was widely approved, and this, too, was in tune with the spirit of the times. Acts of Parliament prohibiting at least the worst exploitation of children were, by then, old history but in the late 1880s, when reforms were crowding each other out of the public's notice, the education of children still held an important place. Side by side with the popular current conception of the 'girl of the period' – the Rose Leyburn type – the 'child of the period', a self-assured infant, began to appear in *Punch* and other journals with a sense of what was going on.

Writing of children's clothing in the *Woman's World* of July 1888, Mrs Oscar Wilde noticed that dresses of the past, by which she meant fashions of the past, were being adapted to conform to modern ideas. From this it seemed to follow that children, however hygienically dressed, should look a little quaint.

> It is probably owing to artists having turned their attention to matters of dress that we see so many picturesquely dressed children around us. Many of these dresses are historical, and the favourite dress for both boys and girls seems to be the Charles I dress. We have little Cavaliers in plush tunics and knickerbockers with coloured silk sashes and Vandyck collars . . .[27]

Apart from being the Fauntleroy dress this had been worn, of course, by Mrs Haweis's Lionel in the 'seventies and is an example of the efforts to dispense with changes of fashion in favour of something that could be regarded as permanently beautiful. The author of the article, however, did not quite support the Fauntleroy uniform – and it is interesting to discover that it was already so popular when he put it on – for she continues:

> I am glad that plush is rather giving way to rough clothes for children's outdoor dress. Plush is a very beautiful material but besides the fact that there are very common imitations of it, it seems scarcely suitable for the free physical life that is so absolutely necessary for every healthy child.[28]

Nor was plush suitable, though Mrs Wilde may not have realised it at the time, to the new democratic ideas and the East Ending of the thoughtful well-to-do; art serge and linen smocks, although probably never worn by the children of the working-classes, had a pleasing classlessness about them.

The same issue of the *Woman's World* informed its readers that 'the kindergarten costume introduced by the Rational Dress Society should be adopted by all mothers who wish their girls to grow up healthy and happy.'[29] The kindergarten was itself, of course, a new idea and a sign of the times.

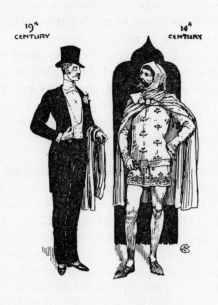

8

The Attack on Tubes

Reforms in the clothing of men had taken a different course. Although it had been agreed since the middle of the 19th century that men's dress was ugly and inconvenient, men as a sex were, unlike women, engaged in no crusade that might have made it desirable for them to change their image.

In the 1850s, long before Dr Jaeger's *Essays* were written, doctors were urging men to wear wool; and in 1851 Dr Beale, among others, had stressed the importance of wearing flannel next to the skin for, 'Woollen promotes transpiration'. The story of the commanding officer who had kept his troops fit in a hot climate, and therefore victorious in their campaigns, by insisting on woollen body-belts, was repeated in most medical hand-books; but the design of men's outer clothing was not, on the whole, mentioned at all.

Dr Jaeger himself, however, wrote far more forcibly about men's dress than women's which he considered rather less evil. What he had to say about the urgent reforms in men's dress involved redesigning their outer garments as well as changing the fabrics worn beneath. In view of his abhorrence of draughts, Dr Jaeger naturally disapproved of trousers:

> The indignant contempt which I have long felt for the mode in which men are condemned by modern artificiality to clothe their legs has been accentuated by reading a pathetic account of a ball lately held at the Tübingen University ... a large number of the ladies were forced to sit inactive ... because the men lacked the inclination to dance ... I maintain that, given equally good constitution and health every lady can wear out her partner, and the reason for this (for men) ignominious fact, is that the costume of males is much more prejudicial to the physical energy and power of performance, and therefore much less healthy than that of females.[1]

Dr Jaeger, in ascribing the weariness of the men at the dance at Tübingen to trousers, assumed that all the women wore, beneath their skirts, closed knickers which fitted round the knee and therefore precluded the ascent of any draughts.

After tracing the evolution of trousers – they were all right as long as they were cross-gartered – Dr Jaeger saw in the 16th-century fashion, which divided hose from breeches, a 'retrogression', hygienically speaking, because 'the knee breeches soon came to be worn wide, and in consequence were insanitary; moreover the garter and the overlapping of breeches and stocking impeded the equal distribution of blood in the leg'.[2]

For modern trousers Dr Jaeger had nothing but contempt, calling them, among other things, unaesthetic monstrosities:

> By leaving the legs too cold, while keeping the abdomen too warm, i.e. by causing a faulty distribution of the blood, and,

consequently, an unequal nourishment of those parts of the body, the modern trousers are responsible for the sparrow-like legs and protruding stomachs, which are so common with men.[3]

In Dr Jaeger's view it was essential to change to stockings and breeches, both of them knitted or made of stockinet, and preferably undyed; or, as a less hygienic alternative, dyed with indigo. Knee-breeches were certainly better than trousers, but 'the hygienically correct ideal would be breeches of stockinet cloth, fitting closely to the shape of the leg, such as were worn in the Middle Ages, not flapping about the boot (or shoe) but, on the contrary, enclosed by it'.[4] Here Dr Jaeger evidently had what are now called 'tights' in mind.

Answering in advance the criticism that such closely fitting long breeches would reveal the sorry shape of the legs of most men, Dr Jaeger confidently promised that under his System they would soon improve. The breeches must be held up by Sanitary Woollen Braces and accompanied by the Sanitary Woollen Shirt. Except in cases of ill-health, old age, or extreme thinness, under-pants were undesirable and instead the back, or tail, of the shirt should be drawn between the legs and fastened to the front by means of a safety-pin. Dr Jaeger, though totally rejecting any vegetable fibres in the clothing, did not regard metal as in any way insanitary.

The fastening of the shirt itself should be not in front but on one shoulder, and over it should be worn the coat, made in stockinet and without any trace of linen or cotton fibre. It should be double-breasted and never worn unbuttoned though it could be removed altogether when the weather was sufficiently warm. [37] Like the Sanitary Woollen Coat itself, the sleeves should fit closely and any gap at the wrist should be closed, 'by webbings, to prevent the injurious effects of a current of air ascending between the coat-sleeve and the shirt . . . . a pocket depending from the belt and made of the same material, as worn in the Middle Ages by men would be best'.[5] In the pocket would be the Sanitary Woollen Handkerchief, which, if made of cashmere, would be beautifully soft and smooth, warm,

comfortable and *wholesome-smelling*. Gloves would naturally be
made of wool.

Head-coverings presented rather more problems. It would be
better to wear none at all but this would prove very difficult in
view of changes of climate. There must certainly be no cotton
fibre either as lining or trimming; in summer a straw-hat
(undesirable because vegetable) could be replaced by one
made of plaited horsehair. Dr Jaeger admitted that soft hats
could not be worn on all occasions, so he had spent considerable pains in producing a really black top-hat which could
be dyed only with pure indigo, free from the logwood which
was usually required to produce a good black. For ordinary
occasions the hygienically superior soft undyed hat should be
chosen.

For his own wear Dr Jaeger had a 'weather-mantle' made in
the form of a South American poncho:

> On the inner side of the hinder portion a girdle is fixed which
> may be fastened round the waist either under or over the
> front portion. In the former case the front portion hangs free,
> and one extremity of it can be thrown over the shoulder
> forming the artistic fold of a Roman toga. If, however, the
> front portion is secured by fastening the girdle round it, one
> extremity of the hinder portion may be tucked in under the
> girdle, so as to give an artistic fold, either on the right or on
> the left.[6]

While it is agreeable to find that at this point Dr Jaeger takes
aesthetics into consideration, it is at the same time surprising,
for the extra folds would inevitably lead to a multiplication of
layers in some areas and hence, surely, to an imbalance in the
distribution of the blood.

It has been noted that at the opening of the International
Health Exhibition Mr Edwin Chadwick had appeared as a
member of the official party, dressed according to Dr Jaeger's
Sanitary Woollen System. It appears that either while he was
actually writing the final version of his *Health Culture* in 1885 or
very soon afterwards, Dr Jaeger extended his ideas on male

Sanitary dress to include a combination garment designed to be worn on the outside; for at some time in the later 1880s the most famous Briton to adopt the Jaeger System, George Bernard Shaw, is reported as wearing this even more extreme form of dress.

Shaw came across the Jaeger theories through an Austrian political refugee, Andreas Scheu, who was earning his living in London by setting up a Jaeger business in the West End. Shaw, then about thirty, apparently needed no persuasion to adopt Dr Jaeger's reformed dress and even went so far as to buy what a biographer, Frank Harris, described as an 'ideally healthy single garment or combination in brown knitted wool, complete from sleeves to ankles in one piece in which a human being resembled nothing but a forked radish in a worsted bifurcated stocking'.[7]

Harris called the Jaeger woollens 'brilliant stockinet cloths', but later referred to Shaw as appearing on the stage to take a call on the first night of the production of his first play, *Widower's Houses*, in 1892, in 'a dazzling suit of silver-grey'. Presumably the pale natural wool which Dr Jaeger advocated must have looked 'brilliant' in contrast to the black habitually worn by the men of the time, since it cannot have been dyed. In his forked-radish suit Bernard Shaw walked, according to his biographers, from Tottenham Court Road to the Marble Arch without interference; but although he continued to wear Jaeger suits cut in a more or less normal way, he does not appear to have persisted in the wearing of the external combinations. G. K. Chesterton, writing about Shaw in 1910, gives an endearing picture of his appearance:

> . . . his costume has become a part of his personality; one can come to think of the reddish-brown Jaeger suit as if it were a sort of reddish-brown fur, and was, like the hair and eyebrows, a part of the animal . . . the man is so much of a piece and must always have dressed appropriately. In any case his brown woollen clothes, at once artistic and hygienic, completed the appeal for which he stood; which might be defined as an eccentric healthy-mindedness.[8]

Shaw was frequently photographed wearing what looks like natural coloured wool which in the first decade of the 20th century was represented by brownish rather than whitish wool; and in full length photographs he is seen in not trousers but knee-breeches with stockings, in the approved compromise admitted by Dr Jaeger.

It would have been difficult for anyone with the normal artistic outlook of the later 19th century to see beauty in the two parallel tubes in which men's legs were encased, and it is clear that Dr Jaeger was not the first to prefer breeches to trousers, for they had already been adopted by some of those men who wished to look different from the ordinary urban gentleman. Since knee-breeches had long been worn with gaiters or thick stockings, as sports costume, the aesthetes, although no doubt they laid themselves open to ridicule, were not so conspicuous when they chose to wear knee-breeches as were their feminine counterparts who wore reformed dress. [39, 40, 55] Intellectuals who had worn breeches in the 'seventies merely found themselves in company not only with athletes who specialised in certain sports but with those who attended functions at Court where knee-breeches were a part of correct dress.

In wearing knee-breeches for his first American lecture tour in 1881, therefore, Oscar Wilde had chosen something which was very close to levée dress but the similarity would probably have passed unnoticed in the United States, which preferred its diplomats not to wear a uniform that might have been royal in origin.

In 1893 there appeared the first number of the Journal of the Healthy and Artistic Dress Union with the title *Aglaia* and with a title-page designed by Henry Holiday in the best artistic taste of the time. [41] *Aglaia* was a very different publication from the modest *Gazette* of the Rational Dress Society, but copies of it are exceedingly difficult to find. It announced that the Healthy and Artistic Dress Union had been founded in July 1890 (a year after the demise of the *Gazette* and when the *Woman's World* also ceased to appear), for the propagation of sound ideas on the subject of dress, and requested the reader to *nota bene* that the Vice-Presidents 'support the H & A D U on the express understanding conveyed in the "Introduction" that the Union aims at sound education and discourages personal singularity in dress'.

The Vice-Presidents included Sir Arthur Blomfield ARA, Lady Mary von Hugel, Mrs Louise Jopling, and G. F. Watts; Henry Holiday's name appears as one of the two men on the Executive Committee. The Healthy and Artistic Dress Union owned a small library of about twenty books and hoped to add to it – it gave their names, headed by *Studies in Greek Art* by Jane Harrison. Among the others are those of Mrs Haweis and Mrs Balling and, of course, Dr Jaeger's *Health Culture*. The second number of *Aglaia* announced that in the following November a paper would be read on 'Pernicious Advertisements'.

Aglaia was elegantly produced, with good illustrations and, at a shilling, must have been aimed at a fairly prosperous readership. The second number included an article by Henry Holiday on Men's Dress, partly reprinted from an earlier article by him in the *English Illustrated Magazine*. Holiday pointed out that the modern tailors' ideal could never be achieved:

> It is useless for tailors to draw gentlemen in trousers without a crease, it is useless for them to supply 'trouser-stretchers' to efface every night all evidence of their ever having clothed a human limb during the day; so long as human limbs are formed on one principle and garments on another the result will be a failure . . . The Tailors must find a Utopia for their tubes; in this fallen world they are a failure – Heaven be praised![9]

Holiday illustrated his articles by comparative drawings, one of a group of late 15th-century men taken from Pinturrichio's frescoes in the *Libreria* in Siena, and the other of men and boys of the 1890s labelled, 'a long way from Pinturrichio'; and, on the next page, three comparative drawings, the *Apollo Belvedere*, a man in city dress, and a comfortably clothed modern man wearing a soft shirt with an unstarched turned-down collar, a scarf-tie, a loose coat, and knee-breeches. The knee-breeches are supported not by braces but a belt, the hair is bushy and long enough to reach the nape of the neck. [42, 43]

Some space and one or two drawings were devoted to Greek dress which Holiday regarded as perfection, and he then returned to the modern ideal, starting with natural leather brown boots with plenty of room for the toes, and, since the 'leg is a wonderful piece of construction'[10] advocated knee-breeches as a fairly good second-best to medieval hose:

> It will be seen that with the knickerbocker we entirely lose the beauty and interest of the knee. We get the lower leg it is true, but its swelling curves, which are so full of charm and significance when they are seen gradually developing from the firmly-knit articulation of the knee, lose nearly all this interest when they emerge from the bulging form of the knickerbocker.[11]

Knickerbockers had lately come into fashion for country and sports' wear.

Holiday regarded cloth as having a beauty and a character of its own,[12] but the tube gave no scope for the rich and massive folds which were one of its chief beauties; softness and pliability were desirable and, starting with the shirt, should replace the unbending stiffness of breastplate, handcuffs, and collar which were, 'as badges of our servitude to the tyrant Fashion'. As for the coat, the Norfolk jacket was a move in the right direction but its pleats were too formal, and 'we may hope that something more in the nature of a blouse for country wear may be adopted in time'.[13]

And the present overcoat, again, was nothing but a tube and would be greatly improved by the addition of some soft folds as well as a cape such as that attached to the Ulster but long enough to be of some practical use. After a few words on evening dress, Henry Holiday concluded:

> There must be in society a large number of people who individually would not regard it as a proof of insanity that a man should dress like a rational being. If all such would each in their separate circles make the proposition to such friends as were likely to be sympathetic on the subject, we should

have a number of nuclei formed of groups of people whose informal gatherings would be enlivened by their pleasant and reasonable form of attire, and it is probable that the obvious advantage of the change would soon lead to a wide extension of the practice, until in an educated society the miserable old heap of dingy tubes, meaningless angles, and stiff cardboard might find itself in a despised minority.[14]

In these gentle, tentative words one almost imagines one hears the Aunt conversing with her progressive nieces in the 1860s.

Although Henry Holiday followed Dr Jaeger in commending close-fitting knee-breeches as a reasonably good alternative to 'mediaeval' hose, the loose jacket hanging in graceful folds from the shoulders with no fastening at all in front would have been labelled by Dr Jaeger insanitary. Unlike Dr Jaeger with his forked-radish, Henry Holiday never suggested a return to mediaeval hose, however artistic they might have been as clothing.

For the third issue of *Aglaia*, Walter Crane wrote and illustrated an article on the Progress of Taste in Dress, related especially to education in art. After discussing the design of women's clothes he spoke of some of the problems facing men. Since, for instance, it was agreed that knee-breeches, silk stockings, and buckled shoes were more becoming than tubes, these could be adopted by ordinary citizens; but what, in that case, would become of 'the Cabinet Minister at Court, my Lord Mayor, Mr Speaker and other notabilities?'[15] These complexities seemed 'to convince one that the costume is really controlled by the forms of social life, condition, occupation, rank, general tradition, sentiment and sense of fitness, so that we can only expect great changes in the outside of life when corresponding changes are affecting the inside – the foundation, constitution and moral tone of society'.[16]

Here indeed is the crux of the problem which faced dress-reformers in the 'nineties. Beauty, continued Crane,

is inseparably associated with love, and . . . we cannot expect to get beauty at any price if, while arranging an elaborate system of art education on the one hand, we allow ourselves to destroy its sources in nature, in the beauty of our own land, by ruthless destruction or vulgarisation now too common.[17]

That these sentiments could be uttered in an article on the reform of the design of dress is an indication of the changes that were taking place.

Soon after the beginning of the 'nineties, indeed, it is clear that while East Ending continued among those who had taken it seriously from the beginning, the eyes of the fashionable social groups which had merely regarded it as a modish amusement began to be attracted by a new and glittering temptation – a late-born descendant of the idea that vice was absolutely more attractive than virtue. The fact that Swinburne had seen vice as active while virtue was palely passive was over-looked, and the new generation put out the idea that on the contrary, virtue was over-active and a bore. Almost overnight it ceased to be fashionable to East End.

Walter Crane illustrated his article on dress by some designs for artistic clothing for women and children, no longer of first interest as the reformer's target, and then added a splendid drawing of two well-built picturesquely clothed specimens of working-class men – a trawlerman in a sou'wester, knitted jersey, and boots, and a road-mender in corduroys, his shirt-sleeves rolled up and the sleeves of his coat knotted round his neck. Crane was an active Socialist and these were his new heroes. He followed them by another drawing of two contrasting types of dress, a Piccadilly Johnny in tails and a monocle and a relaxed bearded man in a dress labelled '14th century'. [Headpiece Chapter 8]

Aglaia itself was not quite ready to step along with Crane's political ideas. It followed, instead, Henry Holiday's suggestion for a new type of evening dress for men and reproduced an illustration of three men wearing it – one of them an idealised young Oscar Wilde, another a likeness of Walter Crane [48]. The suits they wore – soft shirts, cutaway coats, knee-breeches – were, the text suggested, to be made in velveteen:

The colour would be left to the taste of the wearer, but it would probably be discreet to begin with very quiet colours, such as brown, purplish or bronze, or russet, or deep quiet greens, or black.[18]

The stockings, it was suggested, should be of the same colour as the velveteen. Knee-breeches, the text pleaded, were really not unfamiliar in these days of cycling:

We venture to hope that wherever a few friends agree to support each other in adopting this costume, they will be conscious of making a step towards better taste without feeling that they are wearing anything very strange ... It is not suggested that any one should wear this dress under circumstances which would make it eccentric but at home, or in gatherings of a few friends who are in sympathy with the movement, there would be no such risk, and if one or two who were present did not wear the dress they might be influenced to make the experiment themselves ... The cost of the velveteen is about six guineas, or if lined with silk, seven guineas.[19]

Apart from these articles in *Aglaia* not very much more was ever heard of these particular suggestions in the direction of the reform of men's dress; they came, as has been suggested, at a moment when the minds of most progressively minded people were turned in another direction and one which was not disposed to place much emphasis on occasions demanding evening dress.

A poignant manifestation of this spirit was a book published in 1891, William Morris's *News from Nowhere*, a Utopia perhaps vaguely suggested by Samuel Butler's *Erewhon* of 1871 but very different in character. The action of the book takes place in the first decade of the 21st century and the author is transported, Rip van Winkle-like, into that moment in the future, in the new London. The book makes particularly harrowing reading now for, the workers' revolution having taken place in 1952 and the ugly buildings having been destroyed soon after, the new London had been rebuilt as a garden city, set in woodlands and free from any trace of dust or dirt. Almost all the 'ugly' buildings had been removed – the British Museum, St Paul's and the Houses of Parliament (used as a dung-market) were exceptions to serve as a foil for the new. Of one of these new buildings,

> One can say little more than that it seemed to me to embrace the best qualities of the Gothic of northern Europe with those of the Saracenic and Byzantine, though there was no copying any of these styles. On the other, the south side . . . was an octagonal building with a high roof not unlike the Baptistry in Florence in outline.[20]

From this new London of the early 21st century all commerce had disappeared and there was no more money; the whole male population and those females who felt like it worked to please the community and therefore themselves. The visitor from the 19th century (writing in the first person) became aware that he must have been in Chiswick where he encountered, on the Thames, a waterman who

> was dark-haired and berry-brown of skin, well-knit and strong, and obviously used to exercising his muscles, but with nothing rough or coarse about him, and clean as might be. His dress was not like any modern work-a-day clothes I had seen, but would have served very well for a picture of fourteenth century life: it was of dark blue cloth, simple enough, but of fine web and without a stain on it. He had a brown leather belt round his waist, and I noticed that its clasp was of damascened steel beautifully wrought. In short, he seemed to be like some specially manly and refined young gentleman, playing waterman for a spree, and I concluded this was the case.[21]

It was not, of course. The clothes of the waterman corresponded more or less to those of the 'fourteenth century' man drawn for *Aglaia* as a contrast to the opera-hatted dude. William Morris's waterman must have been wearing the mediaeval hose which Henry Holiday had longed for but dared not propose and

in which Bernard Shaw had walked from Tottenham Court Road
to the Marble Arch. In fact, Walter Crane's working-men were
nearer to the unattainable ideal, and although it took nearly
another thirty years before earnest young readers of the *New
Statesman* could wear corduroy trousers and a rough jacket, the
way was opened to them by dress-reformers of the 1890s.

William Morris himself wore with his inevitable indigo-dyed
suit a deep-blue shirt. The navy-blue suit gradually became, in
the early days of the 20th century, the Sunday wear of every
British working man who could afford one, and the daily wear
of those of the middle-classes whose employers were liberal
enough to allow them to discard the dying frock-coat and
silk hat. The indigo suit eventually found its way into Bernard
Shaw's *Caesar and Cleopatra* in which Brittanus wears dark-blue
woad, the uniform, it is explained, of his country.

Trousers did not, of course, disappear and breeches remained
only as Court dress and cycling and sports clothing. Dr Jaeger's
undyed stockinet was not generally adopted – in pressing it on
his disciples he had been alone. It was, in any case, not so much
a sanitary reality as a symbol of democracy that reformers
wanted in the 'nineties, and this was supplied to some extent by
tweeds, hand-woven by British Celts and made in colours that
were, or could have been, produced by vegetable dyes. Although
few working-class men wore such hand-woven tweeds (they
naturally preferred the more refined surface of serge), they
looked serviceably rough and unaristocratic; in point of fact
they soon passed, following the immutable law, into high
fashion as the country wear for gentlemen and remained as the
normal dress of many artists for a long time.

Many of the ideas put forward in the International Health
Exhibition and urged by humanitarians and by some members
of the medical profession appealed to those men who pinned
their faith to the particular and numerous versions of Marxist-
Socialism which were spreading through Britain in the 1890s.
Among these ideas were dress reform, vegetarianism (practised
by saints and reformers since the beginning of recorded customs), the refusal to wear furs and most feathers, and the dislike
of highly polished fine-grained woods; silver, pewter and

copper were preferred to costly and symbolic gold, and enamel-work to precious stones. The taste was conveniently at hand to greet the appearance of the art style named 'nouveau'.

The combination of these characteristics was exactly what the newest generation – children while their parents were engaged in the reforms of the earnest 'eighties – found intolerable. It is doubtful whether Oscar Wilde, who had remained a prophet for some sections of society, still kept his sage-green handkerchief in the 'nineties and, if he wore a green carnation, it was in a well-cut black morning coat [46, 49]. Both Aubrey Beardsley and the sensitive young Graham Robertson dressed in the height of Philistine fashion; the *Yellow Book* had no truck with the Socialism of Morris and Walter Crane.

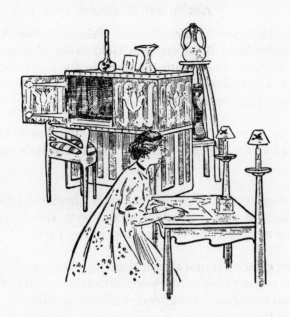

9

Socialist Gowns

The two ideals – beautiful dress and healthy dress – were still an issue in the journal *Aglaia* (which survived for only three numbers) in the autumn of 1894. Among the advertisements, Messrs Capper Son & Co. Ltd illustrated the 'Athenian' Gown (recommended by both the *Gentlewoman* and the *Queen*). The Athenian Gown was described by the advertisers [51]:

A classical Grecian Tea-Gown in soft French crêpons, with hand-made Border of Gold Braid and very full soft Crêpe de Chine sleeves; the whole easily adjusted, and forming an exceedingly graceful and artistic Gown for evening wear.

Made in Ivory White, Apricot, Primrose, Eau de Nil,
Turquoise Blue, Black etc with Gold Braid, also in White,
Pale Grey or Black, with Silver Braid for slight mourning
£4.4.0 ... Square Neck and Crêpe de Chine Sleeves removable on separate bodice, 5/s extra.[1]

Side by side with Athenian Gown, Capper Son & Co. Ltd
presented an engraving of Capper's *Csandco* Hygienic Knickers
[50],

This Artistic and Hygienic garment is scientifically cut so as
to admit of perfect freedom to the body either Walking,
Riding or Sitting; no strain or drag in any part.[2]

At first glance it would appear that these knickers, for which
the 19th century's use of the word 'artistic' seems to have been
somewhat stretched, were intended as cycling breeches; but an
article in the first number of *Aglaia*, called The Distribution of
Weight in Clothing, shows that this is not so, for in discussing
underclothing the author emphasises the inconvenience of
petticoats:

Skirts have the great disadvantage of encasing both lower
limbs together in a common sheath. This is a much colder
form of dress, and one much more difficult to walk in than
some form which clothes each leg separately ... Divided
skirts have many draw-backs in common with petticoats, but
rather loose knickerbockers fastening with a couple of
buttons by a shaped band below the knee, are perfectly
satisfactory. With these, long black gaiters can be worn out-
of-doors. If the knickerbockers are well-fitted round the hips
they do not usually need any other attachment, but they may
be made to button on a bodice .... or they may be cut in one
piece up to the neck as a combination garment. For the
material of these knickerbockers, or combinations, there is a
black stockinette stuff made for riding trousers, which answers
very well, or of cloth to match the dress, or they may be made
of navy-blue serge ...[3]

Capper & Co., claimed that their knickers were 'scientifically cut and made in fine coating cloth with a removable flannel lining'.

Presented as they are, side by side with the Athenian Gown, it is difficult not to imagine, as may well have been intended, that the one was designed to be worn beneath the other, which, in comparison, makes E. W. Godwin's suggestion that Greek dress was only suitable in England if worn over woollen combinations seem almost elegant.

It is also difficult not to imagine that both Walter Crane and Henry Holiday must have shuddered at the engraving which presented the Athenian Gown, an ill-favoured offspring of their creative efforts to bring back the grace of the clothing of the Greeks [51]. Much nearer to the ideal which they shared were versions of the fashions of the beginning of the 19th century which were, in the middle of the 'nineties, enjoying a short vogue – both as picturesque versions of the normal high-fashion and as clothing for characters in many genre paintings. *Aglaia's* first number included a short piece on this fashion, illustrated by some attractive drawings, as to how it could be made to comply with really artistic dress. All the designs could be charming, and the author suggested 'pale apricot gauze over a salmon or a warm pink dress, or a pale primrose gauze over a turquoise or a sea-green silk would be very tender and beautiful. As gauze can be had shot, yet more subtle harmonies can be obtained; a delicate embroidery on the edges of the gauze, and a judicious colour in the trimming of the yoke . . . . would give an opportunity for increasing the interest of the harmony of colour'.[4]

The modern mind naturally recoils from the suggestion that navy-blue knickers lined with flannel could be worn beneath these delicate 'Empire' dresses; even Dr Jaeger, however, had allowed that for ceremonial occasions, provided wool was worn underneath, some other fabric was admissible on top.

Praise for the Athenian Gown from both the *Queen* and the *Gentlewoman* indicates that at least some forms of artistic dress were considered worth distributing on a commercial basis. The appearance of a third-hand Greek dress during the revival of the 'Empire' style shows that even in the 1890s Greek dress retained its appeal. It was chosen, for instance, by George du Maurier (whose mocking observation of artistic extravagances had missed very little over the previous twenty years) as the costume in which his Trilby made her début on the London concert platform [53], while Watts, reappearing in a brief article in *Aglaia*, referred once more to the 'noble form of the head' as exemplified by the Venus of Milos. *Aglaia*, which had undertaken not to support personal singularity in dress hastened to assure its readers that the 'Helen of Troy' and the 'Fair Rosamund' as drawn (probably by Holiday) in its first issue, had not been intended as fashion-plates nor 'as our suggestion for a walking-dress to be worn in Regent Street. They are included in *Aglaia* as reminders of what the unspoiled human figure is, how supple and full of life and grace in every movement, and to show how lovely drapery can be when that grace is "made manifest" in it'.[5]

In the same number the ruination of the human figure was the subject of the first of a series of long articles by Dr Wilberforce Smith, who will be remembered as having attacked the wearing of corsets in the *Woman's World* of 1889. Now, writing of Corset Wearing; the Medical side of the Attack, he referred in a footnote to the surgeon, Mr Adaine, who had participated in the British Association's debate on corsets that had so disturbed the Rational Dress Society.

Dr Wilberforce Smith had measured a considerable number of erector ridges of the torsoes of a variety of women including those of five Indian ayahs who had never worn corsets; their measurements and the curve of their backs he had found admirable, whereas English girls

> if dressed in the usual manner, will, like every budding girl within the pale of civilisation, be found to have these muscles of the back partly withered. It is quite otherwise with the few brave women who really abstain from corsets, and from such substitutes as strongly-boned bodices ... the Healthy and Artistic Dress Union invokes *Aglaia* to teach her weaker

sister, Fashion, that health and beauty must be according to truth.[6]

Among the 'few brave women' who abstained from corsets was Mrs Hubert Bland, poetess, author of novels and short stories, and later to become famous as E. Nesbit, author of books for children. In about 1884, when she was twenty-six, she had declared:

> ... I have *cut my hair off* !!!!!! I retain the fringe but at the back it is short like a boy's ... It is *deliciously* comfortable ... I have also taken to all-wool clothing which is also *deliciously* pleasant to wear.[7]

Right at the end of the 'eighties, E. Nesbit was remembered as still wearing her short hair:

> She was quite unlike any woman I had ever seen, with her tall, lithe, boyish-girl figure, admirably set off by her plain 'socialist' gown, her short hair and her large vivid eyes ...[8]

Her 'socialist gown' was the descendant of the PreRaphaelite dress, with full sleeves and folds which ran right down to the hem from the neck. Laurence Housman did a drawing of her playing tennis in it in the 'nineties, by which time it had been approached closely enough by current fashion to look, in its simpler versions, 'socialist', and no longer in any of its forms rebelliously aesthetic.

Throughout the 'nineties, strictly fashionable dress demanded a waist which was as small, if not smaller than any that had preceded it; but even for women who were antagonistic or indifferent to reforms in dress there had appeared garments for wearing in the country, in the morning in town, or informally at home at any time, which did not require tightly laced stays. It was among these less formal garments that the minor fashion for a high-waisted dress first appeared: the dress that could be modified in one direction into something that looked rather Greek (as illustrated in *Aglaia*), in another into a crisper version with a Kate Greenaway air and, strange partnership, in a third could be hardened into the dress, little-girlish in shape but not in implication, that Aubrey Beardsley occasionally used to clothe his infernal half-sisters of the Greenaway innocents. [57]

These variations and hybrids which sprouted fairly vigorously in the soil of the *haute couture* were, before very long, to vindicate Dr Wilberforce Smith for, by 1908, corsets were completely discarded by the most advanced French designers; the following year they had disappeared from all the Paris shows and they were to remain absent from high fashion for well over half a century, if not considerably longer.

As the fashionable dress of women began to include some garments that could be regarded as reasonably 'hygienic', so the attention of reformers was turned more and more to the question of the health, upbringing, education and dress of children. Walter Crane devoted an article,[9] illustrated by himself, to their dress in the number of *Aglaia* which also included an advertisement for a girls' boarding-school [65]. This school would have both astonished and appalled even the most progressive doctors of the middle of the 19th century who had been pioneers in urging schools to provide girls with a more healthy and active life. Its advertisement ran:

Rational Education for Girls
Suffield Park, Cromer.
Ethical and Moral Training are substituted for so-called 'religious' teaching.
The Education of the Body, both for health and skill, is systematically carried out under the care of a specially trained Health Mistress.
Manual work has its proper place in the School Curriculum.

Competition is absent.

For particulars as to Terms, Methods &c., apply to the Principal, Miss H. Clark.[10]

Cromer, on the east coast of England is, of course, particularly bracing; those English girls who were sent there or to other schools of the kind were likely to have emerged very different creatures from their grandmothers. Suffield Park evidently felt it unnecessary to inform the reader of its attitude to cultivated behaviour, the arts or, in fact, any aspect of its academic teaching.

Whether the girls who went to Suffield Park wore artistic dress would be difficult to ascertain but it is reasonable to suppose that they did, since such clothes were being made commercially by the middle of the 1890s and not only by Liberty's. Almost all the dresses for little girls designed by Walter Crane were embroidered, and from the beginning of the 'nineties until the outbreak of the First World War, when it disappeared, the mark of aesthetic rather than merely comfortable dress was its embroidery. The use of embroidery at this particular moment is significant. All the crafts were rapidly dying and hand-work was becoming precious but, even more important, embroidery provided a means of embellishment not only at very little cost apart from the work itself but at what could be seen to be very little cost. And it could be done at home. Linen or wool enriched with embroidery in silk, fitted well into the spirit of the time – simple materials made beautiful by labour. It had been a part of William Morris's dream in 1891, for the classless inhabitants of his utopian *Nowhere* pursued their arcadian tasks in lovely clothes:

> They were making hay busily now in the simple fashion of the days when I was a boy ... the majority of these were young women clad in light woollen mostly gaily embroidered in bright colours. The meadow looked like a gigantic tulip bed because of them.[11]

Although the adjective PreRaphaelite as applied to dress had disappeared from the vocabulary of the 'nineties, characteristic PreRaphaelite puffed sleeves had been taken over, as we have seen, by high fashion and were used without especial mention [56]. Artistic dress, however, survived, though it was changing both its function and its station in life. When it was discussing women's dress *Aglaia* had been mainly concerned to modify and adapt those designs of the conventional fashion which could suit its purpose.

Artistic dress, where it did survive, was no longer a prerogative of the thoughtful well-to-do for, by the end of the century, all over England latter-day Candidas in country parsonages had adopted the current version. Made in simple stuffs, smocked and in other ways embroidered, it was a sign that they and their husbands – emancipated from the fox-hunting clergy of the past who had dined regularly at the Squire's table – favoured the pastoral life with a leftish outlook and supported local debates and University Extension lectures which might attract the working classes to interest themselves in local and even national government [52]. For similar reasons artistic dress found its way into many of the progressive schools where it was not only worn by the pupils, children of the prosperous, but also by members of the staff. Especially it was favoured by those mistresses who were responsible for the arts and found it increasingly difficult to hold their own against the new athletic women of the turn of the century.

Long after women who fought for Women's Rights [59] had abandoned the attempt to stem the course of fashion, and when aristocratic aesthetes had grown so elderly that any remnants of intensity they still practised could only have been regarded as personal eccentricities, artistic dress emerged as a *lingua franca* among women of the middle and working classes who had read William Morris and who followed Robert Blatchford[12] and his colleagues in the *Clarion* week by week. In its first issue, which had appeared on December 12th 1891, Blatchford had described the nature of the *Clarion* in his leading article:

The policy of the *Clarion* is a policy of humanity; a policy not of party, sect or creed, but of justice, of reason and mercy.

Edited with flair rather than science, the *Clarion* gathered into its weekly pennyworth contributors of wildly various talents and views, but stuck to its policy of humanity. One of the numerous manifestations of Socialism and socialist groups, it was designed to be read by anybody, but it was, in fact, largely read by working-class people who encountered for the first time literature, art and music as well as justice, reason and mercy. In 1907 Robert Blatchford published his own Utopia, *Sorcery Shop*. Unlike William Morris, writing sixteen years earlier, he found it difficult to devise a dress for his happy Utopians (they lived in Manchester which Morris has swept away as unfit to survive). By this time the gothicism of Morris was out-of-date but the ideal of simple clothing made of hand-woven stuffs and trimmed with embroideries, still survived.

Worn with a tweed or a dark-blue suit, a cloth cap and a red tie were the sartorial signs of a masculine Socialist at the end of the 19th century. Far too bright to be worn as a part of the normal dress of the period, the red tie was adopted as a political badge by artists, writers and some men sufficiently rich or high-born to be able to ignore the conventions. Apart from such people, and some socialistically-minded workers on the factory floor, members of the male population who depended for their living on the good-will of an employer had to reserve the red tie for week-ends.

The last chapter of a book on one of the narrowest aspects of fashion is not the place to discuss the wider implications of this curious human phenomenon, which penetrates not only every artifact devised by man but also his attitude both to his own creations and to the natural world. Attempts by a small and passionate group to arrest the course of fashion could not have succeeded, and by the end of the 19th century that particular struggle had been virtually abandoned. Its last tiny efforts will be referred to later. By the end of the 'nineties those who wore a kind of dress that had artistic or democratic pretensions wore it to proclaim their personal aesthetic or political standpoints and not their disapproval of changing fashions in dress as such.

Whether garments of the kind that have been discussed in this book could be, or could ever have been, legitimately labelled *artistic* has, of course, nothing to do with the question. It is important to make this clear because, as an ideal, beauty was not set up only in the period which was attacking fashion as a concept. Both before the era of the attack and after it certain clothes which could reasonably be considered to be works of art were worn both in fiction and in life by individual men and women. Samuel Richardson visualised his Clarissa Harlowe as being abducted in such a dress and lingered lovingly over his description of it. Mrs Delany saw two actual dresses on different occasions and wrote to her sister about their rococo embroidery which, from her account, would put them into the category of – say – a fine piece of Bow or a ceiling-painting by Angelica Kaufmann. Millais did a drawing of Effie Ruskin wearing a splendid, strange, embroidered garment and a necklace of wild convolvulus blossoms; and he painted his own children in frocks which, while they conformed to the current fashion, were at the same time original in composition and ornament. There are indications that the same kind of thing went on in 15th-century Florence. These single garments strike no attitudes; they show only that ephemeral things such as clothes, paper fans, and fireworks can occasionally be works of art.

So laborious a statement would be unnecessary but for the fact that rather more examples of clothes of this kind seem to have been recorded in the 'nineties and the early years of the 20th century than seemed usual at other periods [60, 61, 62]. The Belgian artist, Henry van der Velde, who began as an exponent of *l'Art nouveau* and moved into *Jugendstil*, designed unique dresses [62]. A good many beautiful clothes appeared in Germany and Holland at about the same time – expensive, fashionable, and produced not as models but as single pieces. From Paris itself there emanated some startling black and white creations, for which black velvet was cut into decorative designs and laid on to white satin in a style manifestly inspired by the drawings of Aubrey Beardsley and made for one or two women belonging to wealthy American families. It is plain too, from the chic drawings of American girls by Charles Dana Gibson, that descendants of the rather timid aesthetic dresses illustrated in the *Woman's World* of 1889 blossomed into radiant garments that could be worn by young members of the New York smart-set with no other motive than that they looked lovely [54].

Socialist Gowns

The majority of dresses of this kind, worn in the late 1890s and until about 1910, had a high-set waistline which sometimes, but not always, gave them the old-world character which accorded well with the popular genre paintings by Dendy Sadler, an artist whose pictures attracted much admiration at the Royal Academy's Summer Exhibitions, and who clothed his prettily touching scenes in the fashions of the first decade of the 19th century. The love of the sweetly picturesque, the last dying remains of the romantic movement, was still present in some of the clothes of the time, but others which sometimes shared the high-waist, carried with them a Maeterlinkian sigh of woods or floating water-lilies; and still others, as we have seen, made themselves useful to Aubrey Beardsley, who knew all about current fashion.

While all these expensive clothes, real or represented in works of art, could have been labelled artistic, they carried with them no suggestion that their wearers were searching either for a type of dress that would remain permanently 'beautiful' or that they were in any way hygienic. They had nothing in common with the much humbler dresses, home-spun and trimmed with hand-embroidery, which proclaimed their wearers as being both politically sensitive and possessors of good taste.

Contemporary with these lingering vestiges of the reformed dress of the 'seventies and 'eighties came a third type, the commercial, put out chiefly by Liberty's. In 1883 Liberty's issued an illustrated pamphlet called the *Evolution of Costume*. In it were reproduced drawings of some fashions of the first decade of the 19th century and others of the 1830s, neither of them very well understood. Beside each drawing from an original source was an adaptation of the style, suitable for modern wear. The resemblance appears today rather less marked than it probably did when the booklet was published. It is interesting to observe that whereas the proportions of the figures wearing the earlier fashions are more or less normal, those who wear the modern adaptations are shown as very much elongated so that all heads are very small – an important ingredient of beauty according to Watts.

Ten years later, in 1905, Liberty's published a far more ambitious book, illustrated entirely in colour, from which it is clear that picturesqueness still had a market among some of the well-to-do. The collection of clothes illustrated is eclectic: on each page, represented in water-colour, stands a tall young woman, her hair arranged in the current fashion but her dress vaguely reminiscent of some fashion of the past. To avoid any doubt as to the period intended each gown is named: Hera, Iseult [63], Henrietta Maria for instance. All are luxurious, made of silk or velvet, and many are embroidered. Each elegant female stands in a room furnished either in the *art nouveau* style or in a way which mildly recalls an earlier period and one that was fashionable at the time. Most of the objects shown could also, no doubt, be bought at Liberty's. A good many of the dresses, even though embroidered by hand, were very near to the current high-fashion, and all of them could have been worn in any London drawing-room without provoking a smile or a raised eyebrow. They had, perhaps, faintly liberal connotations and might not have been chosen by a Paula Tanqueray; but the presence on the stage of such a woman as the second Mrs Tanqueray, chosen wife of a respected society man, was a far more progressive act on the part of the theatre than the wearing of any dress that could have been ordered from Liberty's.

In 1907 an International Women's Socialist Conference was held in Stuttgart, the home of the early meetings of the Association of German Women, one of which was reported in the first *Woman's World* of 1869. Among the English representatives were Margaret Macmillan, the educational reformer, and Mary Macarthur who was planning to launch a new journal for women the following month. The Women's Socialist Conference was reported at some length in the *Clarion* which noted that the 'First Clap' was provoked by an interesting figure who was 'a French lady with close-cropped hair, tailor-made frock-coat, "masculine" collar and tie and black sailor hat – a perfect gentleman she looked, not to say a gentleman's gentleman'. French women, the article pointed out, stood no chance of being heard in their own country unless they dressed in this way. Frau Lily Brau, a German, 'whose name is so familiar to us, in becoming Liberty frock and flowing veil',[13] disappointed her hearers by speaking in favour of only a limited Adult Suffrage. There were present, it appears, several women who wore the quiet German and Dutch 'reformed dress', which may have been a Continental equivalent to home-spun embroidered clothes worn by their English counterparts or of the plain 'Socialist' dress that E. Nesbit was reported to have worn.

In September 1907 the first number of the journal planned by Mary Macarthur, the *Woman Worker*, the *Clarion's* little sister, appeared with a cover designed by Walter Crane [66]. It ran for a year as a monthly and then became a weekly newspaper. As its name implies it was directed towards working-class women but, like the *Clarion*, its policy was to make no concessions to the fact that its readers might be uneducated except the determination (shared by the *Clarion*) to be readable. On the back cover of the first number appeared an advertisement which read,

> To understand why
> ## WOMEN
> ## SHOULD
> ## VOTE
> Read
> WOMAN: a few shrieks[14]

a reminder that the speech made by Mr Smollett in the House of Commons on the occasion of the second reading of the Women's Disabilities Removal Bill, in 1875, when he had said 'There was an immediate exclamation, I will not call it "a shriek" from the sisterhood',[15] was by no means forgotten.

The second number of the *Woman Worker* included a review of the Clarion Handicraft Exhibition which was, its reviewer said,

> A protest against standardisation ... Instead of the showy jewellery brought home from a holiday at Blackpool or Margate, what sensible working-girl would not prefer some genuine ornament of silver and enamel, made by the designer's own hand, and decorative by its very simplicity, if

such is to be had at a price within her purse . . . The jewellery exhibited is wonderfully effective in spite of the absence of costly material.[16]

This is probably one of the first direct appeals to working-class women on the subject of taste in dress.

Each issue of the *Woman Worker* included an article on some aspect of dress, contributed by a man, Charles E. Dawson, who appeared to have been unfamiliar with earlier controversies on the subject of corsets (or perhaps he presumed that his readers were). In discussing the circulation of the blood, he wrote:

The subject of corset-wearing seems, unfortunately, to be overlooked by the majority of writers of 'Health Notes' or 'Beauty hints' . . . Anyone who has an eye for beauty will see that the Venus de Milo and other fine Greek statues are more beautiful, graceful, and refined in form than the figures one sees in the streets.[17]

The inclusion of the plea 'refined' seems significant in this context – it had not appeared in articles by, for instance, Watts. More original was a statement by the member of Parliament, Leo Chiozza Money who, in an article called 'Daughters of the Gods: ought women to work?' declared:

The strength woman needs to engage increasingly in men's occupations she will gain from the use of her muscles.[18]

Among the articles on the abuses of female labour and the general injustices inflicted on women, the poems by Walter Crane, the passages quoted from Henry James and the reviews of the latest books on political issues, Charles E. Dawson ploughed on with his articles on dress. In the first number of the new series in June 1908, when the paper had become a weekly, he wrote of Fashion and Folly, attacking the new Directoire dresses which were fastened by a tape across the back of the knees inside to give them the required cylindrical line. This was a belated development (for other ideas had intervened) of the 'Empire' revival as a minor fashion in the 'nineties. It was also a convenient device for dispensing with corsets, at last the aim of the Paris *haute couture*. Nor was it altogether without Cubist connotations. Although, however, corsets in the earlier sense were no longer suitable as the basis for a design which was not concerned with reducing the size of the waist, manufacturers were not slow to invent the 'Grecian belting', to be worn above the waist, which, they claimed, would assist the wearer to assume a stance suitable to this revival of a classical style. Grecian belting may, in fact, have been welcomed by women who, determined to follow high fashion, would, nevertheless, have found it difficult to do without the reassuring support that tightly-laced corsets were always said to have provided.

The following week Charles Dawson asked, 'Is This Art?', and advised his readers that 'it is safer to have a costume made of a few shades of one colour – green, brown or blue, for instance – than a dress on the lines of Jacob's coat'; and so the 'blending and shifting hues' of the dress of King Cophetua is handed to the working-classes. A month later Dawson reverted to another theme long forgotten, apparently, in high life:

Fashion will not always rule despotically. As the great upward movement of womanhood broadens and the dawn of woman's consciousness of mighty power grows clear, it will be pleasing to watch its influence upon the 'ladies' papers, and see how long their snobbish twaddle and rag-trade announcements endure.

It is curious to find that the disapproval provoked by the idea that Fashion implies change and change implies Fashion should have loomed so large.

William Morris's *News from Nowhere*, with its belief that an ideal design for dress was simply waiting to be rediscovered, and that once the idealised form of 14th-century clothing had been adopted, no one would want to change it, was still being advertised in the *Clarion* in which, at the moment that Dawson was prophesying the death of Fashion, Robert Blatchford's Utopia, the *Sorcery Shop*, was being serialised. By this time it was too late for anyone as intelligent as Blatchford to believe that society, even though it might revert to the simplicity of a golden age, could do so in mediaeval clothing. He could describe the faces of his Utopians but when he says of a girl that she was a 'symphony in red and brown' it is of her hair and her lips that he speaks: her dress and the dress of the other inhabitants of his Socialist paradise he dared not attempt.

In July of the year 1908, Charles Dawson was bowled over by a new and spectacular young dancer who appeared on the London stage – Maud Allan. Like other contemporary journalists he wrote lyrically about her and, in an article for the *Clarion* called 'The Body Beautiful', he said:

> After studying the masterpieces in the principal galleries of Europe it occurred to her that the lovely dancing figures of Botticelli might by imitation and training be reproduced in living form.

At last, it seems, the struggles towards a reform in dress and the repeated pleas to women to take the best-known Greek Venuses as their models had had their effect. Maud Allan's classical dress was, to judge from her photographs, not particularly convincing but it was nearer the ideals of the reformers than anything that could have been acceptable to audiences at the beginning of the 1880s. Dawson reverted to praise of Maud Allan in several successive articles but six months later he suddenly became much more interested in men's dress:

> As far as men's regulation evening wear is concerned, unimaginative as it is, I do not regard it, like some of our comrades, as the uniform of snobbery so much as the outward and visible sign of an inward and spiritual courtesy ...
> At a recent debate on Socialism Mr Victor Grayson the newly elected MP standing on behalf of the Independent Labour Party for Colne Valley, as a mark of courtesy to his opponent and his audience, appeared in conventional war paint. And the resultant snarling protests of the over-zealous – or hypersensitive – comrades were in as execrable

taste as the vulgar gibes of the upper-middle classes when Mr
Keir Hardie had the courage to go to the House of Commons
in his working clothes.

The young and romantic-looking Victor Grayson was, and
remained, a controversial figure throughout his brief career
in the earlier Socialist days, but Bernard Shaw had encountered
a rather similar difficulty over evening dress.[19] Because he, too,
was a Socialist and one who habitually wore his 'reddish-brown'
hygienic suit, it was assumed that he despised evening dress;
when, therefore, Lord Haldane, sympathetically Liberal,
invited him to meet the Asquiths and Balfour with other Souls,
he suggested that Shaw should come in morning dress. Shaw
rather ruefully concluded that:

There was nothing for it but to dissipate a fortnight's earnings
on a new black suit of the cut then affected by the Labour
appendages of the Liberals in Parliament, in which Shaw
felt, as to the tailless double-breasted jacket, like a ship's
purser at a wedding, and, as to the trousers, like a city
missionary.[20]

Shaw had, as a former music critic, a suit of dress-clothes
which he would willingly have worn, especially as, arriving at
the party, he found that every other male guest was wearing
them. The black, formal Socialist suit had a comparatively short
life and was replaced, after the first war, by a dark-coloured
lounge suit.

For about three years the *Woman Worker* seemed to flourish
and expand; names famous in the Labour movement appeared
week after week in its list of contributors and almost all of them
addressed themselves directly to working-class women. Others,
committed to other journals, wrote under *noms-de-plume*:
'Pandora', for instance, replaced Charles Dawson in November
1908 on,

Dress for the Woman Worker
Avoid Dame Fashion's Dictates.

A young friend of mine has lately brought out a 'Workers' Dress' which is both cheap and artistic. It is made in two or three different styles of plain, good material (of the home-spun type), in various colours; she put a little embroidery on the bodice and the result is delightful.

Here was the first – and the last – tiny step towards Morris's Utopia. How many Workers bought the dress will never be known. Twenty-five years previously the Rational Dress Society had shown examples of Working-women's dress, and offered a prize of £5 for the best. Unfortunately neither the winning example nor any of the others is illustrated in the 1883 catalogue to the Exhibition, but they are most unlikely to have included either embroidery or material of a home-spun type. More significant were the snarling protests that greeted Victor Grayson from his own supporters in the Independent Labour Party when he appeared on the platform in dress clothes, for here were the first indications of a new attitude to dress, a determination to substitute for conventional dress not one which was beautiful or hygienic but one which was classless and, by implication, unceremonious.

The outbreak of the First World War saw the end of deliberate attempts at dress reform in the 19th-century sense, though a recognisable style of dress for women based, apparently, on the Dorelia paintings by Augustus John, was devised and worn by some art students and a few wives of artists and architects until the Second World War. This dress was made with a tight-fitting bodice and a full skirt, gathered into the bodice at the waist and reaching to about the ankles. Since this dress, presumably thought of as more beautiful than the current fashion, arrived at a moment when orthodox dress had itself become very much more comfortable, it must have been worn as a badge proclaiming the taste of the wearer rather than as a protest in favour of something more rational. It was, indeed, a little less rational than fashionable dress, for its skirts were always longer than anything allowed by Paris for daytime wear.

The change from a reformed dress worn as a mission to the unenlightened, to a dress worn as a badge that proclaimed the taste of the wearer may seem subtle but it was important. The reforms urged by champions of the 1870s and early 'eighties were envisaged as changes which would help to bring about a new respect for women, by enabling them to disregard the frivolities of fashion, and a new freedom which would enable them to take their places at work side by side with men – ideals which lingered on, though timidly, in the middle-class *Aglaia* of the 'nineties and the working-class *Woman Worker* of 1908 long after they had been abandoned elsewhere. Bernard Shaw, who travelled with his own woollen sheets, was probably a latter-day supporter of this old cause, much as he would have disliked the label. E. Nesbit who, in her later prosperity, wore flowing artistic gowns, and others who bought the *Hera* and the *Iseult* [63] from Liberty's, may have admired, and indeed worn, clothes very similar to those advocated by Watts; but they wore them, not with missionary zeal, but as expressions of their own tastes and personalities. As women they were already free (apart from a few technical liberties still withheld from them), as were all other English women including those who had no desire to reject conventional dress. If they still had to wait a little while for the Vote it was well on the way.

The attempt to eradicate the pressure of fashion on dress – the most fragile, ephemeral, and intimate building in which man shelters – was the strangest phenomenon in the 19th century's efforts towards dress reform and the least likely to succeed; that the attempt was supported by William Morris but not by Watts is not without its own interest.

Appendixes

Arthur Hugh Clough wrote the poem below in 1845 but it did not receive its title 'A Protest' until his complete works were published by his widow in 1869. Byam Shaw must have felt it to be still appropriate to the position of women in the 1890s and added to its title when he painted 'A Woman's Protest'.

A PROTEST

Light words they were, and lightly, falsely said;
She heard them, and she started, – and she rose,
As in the act to speak; the sudden thought
And unconsidered impulse led her on.
In act to speak she rose, but with the sense
Of all the eyes of that mixed company
Now suddenly turned upon her, some with age
Hardened and dulled, some cold and critical;
Some in whom vapours of their own conceit,
As moist malarious mists the heavenly stars,
Still blotted out their good, the best at best
By frivolous laugh and prate conventional
All too untuned for all she thought to say –
With such a thought the mantling blood to her cheek
Flushed-up, and o'er-flushed itself, blank night her soul
Made dark, and in her all her purpose swooned.
She stood as if for sinking. Yet anon
With recollections clear, august, sublime,
Of God's great truth, and right immutable,
Which, as obedient vassals, to her mind
Came summoned of her will, in self-negation
Quelling her troublous earthy consciousness,
She queened it o'er her weakness. At the spell
Back rolled the ruddy tide, and leaves her cheek
Paler than erst, and yet not ebbs so far
But that one pulse of one indignant thought
Might hurry it hither in flood. So as she stood
She spoke. God in her spoke, and made her heard.

Health, Art & Reason

Appendix 2: ADDITIONAL NOTES ON ILLUSTRATIONS

FRONTISPIECE AND JACKET

Hay Time (The Hayfield). Thomas Armstrong. By courtesy of the Victoria and Albert Museum. Artistic versions of the straight dresses with trains, fashionable very briefly in 1868, after the disappearance of the crinoline and before the acceptance of the Watteau-toilette. This painting was exhibited at the Royal Academy in 1869, so that it must have been painted in that short interval. The dress of the woman holding the child is embroidered with crewel work. (detail)

TITLE PAGE DECORATION

A la Mode a la Mort from *Madre Natura*, 1874. The 'supporter' on the left wears a crinolette.

HEADPIECE CHAPTER 1

A Poser John Leech, Punch 1851 (detail). A young lady wearing a Bloomer asks for the hand of a young man in marriage. For a variation on this, see illustration no. 4.

HEADPIECE CHAPTER 2

Mrs Morris and the Wombat. D. G. Rossetti, pen and ink, British Museum. Jane Morris, in heaven, leads a wombat (William Morris) by a ribbon. Surtees, cat. 607.

HEADPIECE CHAPTER 3

Nature to be perfectly free . . . from *Madre Natura* 1874. A condemnation of the chignon and the Watteau-toilette.

HEADPIECE CHAPTER 4

The Idea! H. R. Howard, Punch 1855 (detail). 'I ax yer pard'n, but yer haven't sich a thing as a lucifer about yer; have yer, missus?': words spoken by a chimney-sweep to a governess in 'strong-minded' dress which is almost identical to that worn by Effie Ruskin in illustration no. 22.

HEADPIECE CHAPTER 5

Fiendish Revenge J. P. Atkinson, Punch (1883). Philistine husband, and wife wearing 'PreRaphaelite' dress. Compare with illustration no. 27. 'Oh George! What are you doing to my beautiful terra-cotta plates?' 'Only practising for the terra-cotta pigeon, my love!'

HEADPIECE CHAPTER 6

Frontispiece to the programme of the Shakespearean Show in the Albert Hall; a part of the Health Exhibition of 1884.

Appendixes

HEADPIECE CHAPTER 7

A Woman's Club. Women of the new independent type wearing fashionable, not reformed, dress. Woman's World 1889.

HEADPIECE CHAPTER 8

A contrast. Modern and Mediaeval Simplicity Walter Crane, Aglaia 1894. The dress of the man on the right which distantly resembles that of a well-known figure in the Spanish Chapel in Florence (already noted by Leighton) belongs to the type envisaged by William Morris when he wrote *News from Nowhere*.

HEADPIECE CHAPTER 9

The Home Made Beautiful R. C. Carter, Punch 1903 (detail). Subtitled 'according to the "Arts and Crafts"', this shows an 'artistic' wife and philistine husband sitting in a room where clearly her taste predominates.

ILLUSTRATION NO. 45: ART IN WHITECHAPEL

The background to the event depicted was described in the Graphic as follows: 'some years ago the idea occurred to ... the Vicar of St Jude's, that ... wealthy owners of pictures might be willing to lend them to be shown to the people whose life is spent amid the dull and ugly conditions of the East End. ... Owners have lent without hesitation ...' The wife of the Vicar was quoted as saying that in 1881 the exhibition, open for nine days, was attended by 9,258 people. In 1882, when it was open for thirteen days including Sundays, 25,776 people came to see it.

Notes

Chapter 1 WOMEN WITH VIEWS *pp. 1–23*

1 According to D. C. Bloomer dress reform was first mentioned in
   1851 when it was said to have been initiated by Mrs Elizabeth Smith
   Miller; Amelia Bloomer wore the dress which was given her name
   in the same year. Bloomer, D. C. pp. 65–67. For Mrs Bloomer's
   description of her dress, id. p. 73.

2 id. p. 72.

3 id. p. 76.

4 id. p. 73. Mrs Bloomer herself called her trousers 'Turkish pantaloons'.

5 *Poetical Broadsides* I p. 41. British Museum 11621.K.4.

6 Reade, *True Love* p. 35.

7 id. p. 61. 'A year after they married, she wanted to give her Bloomer
   to one of the stable-boys. "What, the dress you saved my life in?"
   cried Reginald, "I would not part with it to a Prince, for the price
   of a king's ransom".' p. 63.

8 id. pp. 16, 17.

9 id. p. 38.

10 id. pp. 39–42.

11 id. p. 37.

12 Writing Reade's obituary in the *Fortnightly* in June 1884, W. L.
   Courtney said, '. . . one of his admirers has gone so far as to say that
   he invented the "true woman . . .".'

13 *Edinburgh Review*, July 1862. 'Remains of Mrs Richard Trench;
   being a selection from her Journals Letters and other papers.' Edited
   by her son, the Dean of Westminster. London 1862.

14 *The Owlet Papers*, March 1861, p. 37ff. Heading: The Interior of
   Families. Signed, Zeta.

15 A journal of this name probably already existed but I have not been
   able to trace it. The first issue of the 1868 *Woman's World* appeared in
   May, headed Part I New series.

16 *Woman's World*, October 1868, Part VI, p. 346.

17 *Woman's World*, August 1868, p. 237. From the Earlier Productions of
   Gerald Massey.

18 id. October 1868, p. 361.

19 id. May 1868, p. 26.

19 id. May 1868, p. 26.

20 id. p. 26.

21 id. September 1868, p. 310.

22 id. May 1868, p. 12.

23 id. June 1868, p. 108, '. . . Oh, here comes Ernestine, with Mary,
   Ettie, Amy and Florence', 'A complete Cabinet Council; what is to

be the subject under discussion – the *robe à la queue or robe courte*, Intellectual Culture, or the Woman's Suffrage? . . .'

24 id. July 1868, Fashion Supplement.

25 *The Owl*, 22 April 1868. Article headed, *Heads and Tails*, which began, 'Wigs and Bustles! Wigs were worn in the last century, Bustles in this . . .'

26 id. 6 July 1864, p. 4, 'A Cry from the Ladies' Gallery of the House of Commons. (Dedicated to Sir George Bowyer* by a Modern Lovelace.) *Vide House of Commons, evening sitting, June 30.'

27 *Woman's World*, Vol. II, Part XVI, from Commencement. New series November 1868, p. 64 (the numbering of the parts of WW is somewhat confused). 'Our Gossip. . . . As Byron says, "The world is too much with us . . ."'.

28 *Kettledrum* was issued in a cover similar to that of *Woman's World* but printed in colour instead of monochrome. The first issue was called, Part I, new series, Part XVI, from Commencement.

29 *Woman's World*, November 1868, p. 55.

30 *Kettledrum*, Part XVI, p. 21ff, '. . . The intense realism of the painting is so brave and stern, you will at first think it is all harsh and wrong. . . . You see at a glance from the character of the room that it forms part of one of those cheaply-built villas which spring up in the neighbourhood of our great cities. The furniture is cheap, modern and veneered . . .'

31 id. Part XIX, p. 254.

32 Mill, *Subjection of Women*, pp. 46–47.

33 *Woman's World*, June 1868, p. 121.

34 Combe, Chap. 3.

35 id. Chap. 3.

36 Cook, *Nightingale*, vol. I, p. 195. From the Roebuck Committee Report.

37 Combe, p. 6.

38 id. p. 106.

39 id. p. 182.

Chapter 2 PreRaphaelite Clothing *pp. 24–35*

1 W. Holman Hunt, *PreRaphaelitism and the PreRaphaelite Brotherhood*, vol. I, p. 90.

2 id. p. 138.

3 id. p. 91.

4 id. p. 132.

5 W. Holman Hunt, vol. II, p. 491.

6 id. p. 491. In his biography of his father, Millais' son speaks more strongly, 'Raphael, the idol of the art world, they dared to think, was not altogether free from imperfections. . . . They must go back to earlier times for examples of sound and satisfactory work and, rejecting

the teaching of the day that blindly followed in his footsteps, must take
Nature as their only guide.' Millais, vol. I, p. 49.

7 Reade, *Christie Johnstone*, pp. 76–7
8 W. Holman Hunt, vol. I, p. 137.
9 Millais, vol. I, p. 162.
10 id. p. 141.
11 Roger Smith, *Bonnard's Costume Historique – a PreRaphaelite Source Book* in *Costume*, the journal of the Costume Society, vol. VII, 1973, p. 28ff.
12 Millais, vol. I, p. 94.
13 id. p. 3.
14 W. Holman Hunt, Vol. I, p. 61.
15 There are several drawings of Miss Siddal wearing the same dress and obviously done at the same period; some are dated and some are not. Among them are: Birmingham Museum and Art Gallery no. 260'04 and Cambridge, Fitzwilliam no. 2155.
16 Reproduced in Surtees catalogue.
17 Surtees catalogue nos: 132a, 118, 92.
18 W. Holman Hunt, Vol. I, p. 151.
19 *Aglaia*, 1894, p. 7.
20 Reade, op. cit.

Chapter 3 Grecian Fillets *pp. 36–58*

1 *The Owl*, 16 February 1865. Back page, 'Ondina, or waved jupons, 18s. and 21s. "Let our wives and daughters and their sons' wives and daughters patronise the patent Ondina" – *Punch*. "The dress falls in graceful folds" – *Morning Post*. "Learned in the art of petticoats" – *Le Follet*. E. Philpott, 37 Piccadilly.'
   Id. 20 March 1865. Back page, 'Ebonite Crinolines, 15s. 6d. and 17s. 6d. "Made from Indiarubber, light and graceful" – *Queen*. "Good taste, with an artistic eye" – *Morning Post*. Addley Bourne (late Philpott), 37 Piccadilly.'
2 Paris, Jeu de Paume.
3 *Woman's World*, November 1868, p. 47. Headed 'From the Continent'.
4 Oliphant, *At his Gates*, vol. II, p. 151. Clara was eighteen. Later in the novel (p. 227) we read that Clara, 'contracted her white forehead which was not very high by nature'. The low forehead is a characteristic of Greek sculpture.
5 Limner, p. 11.
6 id. p. 16.
7 id. p. 18.
8 id. p. 30. '. . . French *artistes* or their imitators . . . transform them into far less *natural* creatures than monkeys, as "Girls of the Period".'
9 id. p. 57ff.
10 id. p. 69n.
11 id. pp. 71–3.
12 id. p. 46.

Notes

13 id. p. 80.
14 id. p. 87.
15 id. p. 103.
16 id. p. 112.
17 Wightwick Manor, near Wolverhampton, Staffs. (National Trust).
18 Yonge, *Three Brides*, p. 53.
19 id. p. 155. The Venus de Milo of course has no arms.
20 id. p. 157.
21 id. p. 162.
22 Disraeli, *Lothair*, p. 34.
23 id. p. 100.
24 id. p. 138–139.
25 id. p. 184.
26 *The Owl*, 12 May 1869. 'The Royal Academy'.
27 Oliphant, *Carita*, Vol. II, pp. 229–231.
28 *The Queen*, 5 January 1878. The same issue discussed the 'insipid' lectures given by the American Dr Mary Walker and added, 'While in England she distinguished herself chiefly by the eccentricity of her attire, which was more convenient than picturesque'.
29 James Robinson Planché, Somerset Herald and author of successful plays and pantomimes produced mainly at Drury Lane, published the second volume of his Cyclopaedia in 1878 at the age of eighty-two. The Cyclopaedia of Costume is still a standard work and a source which few, if any later writers on the history of dress, have failed to use.
30 *The Queen*, 5 January 1878. *Art of Dress*, p. 101–106.
31 id. February 1878. *Art of Dress*, p. 108.
32 Howe, *Arbiter of Elegance*, pp. 132 and 133.
33 Haweis, *Art of Dress*, p. 44.
34 id. p. 45.
35 id. p. 46.
36 id. p. 67.
37 id. p. 70.
38 id. p. 120.
39 id. p. 120.
40 Arnold, *Modern Element in Literature*, p. 8.
41 Farrar, *Silence and Voices*, Vol. III, p. 62.
42 Haweis, *Art of Decoration*.

Chapter 4 THE STRONG-MINDED WOMAN *pp. 59–69*

1 Stanton, *Woman Question*, p. 4, Millicent Fawcett on the 'Women's Suffrage Movement'.
2 *The Times*, 9 April 1868, p. 10.
3 Carlyle, Jane, *Letters*, Vol. III, p. 1.
4 Braddon, *Lady Audley's Secret*, Vol. I. p. 259,
5 Burton, *Bodichon*, p. 43.
6 *Saturday Review*, 'Female Suffrage', 28 March 1868.
7 id. 13 June 1868.

8 *The Times*, 9 April 1868, p. 8.

9 *Punch*, 20 April 1868. *Essence of Parliament*, p. 197.

10 id. 20 June, *Essence of Parliament:* Married Women's Property Bill. p. 271.

11 *Hansard*, Wednesday, 7 April 1875, p. 449.

12 id.

Chapter 5 THE EARLY 'EIGHTIES p. *70–88*

1 *Patience*, Act I. Bunthorne.

2 id. Lady Jane.

3 id. Bunthorne.

4 id. Act II. Trio: Duke, Colonel and Major.

5 id. Saphir.

6 Haweis, *Art of Beauty*, p. 221.

7 id. p. 69.

8 id. p. 28.

9 id. p. 25. Chapter headed: Moralities of Dress.

10 Traill/Mann, *Social England*, Vol. 6, p. 596: Literature.

11 id. Stephens, p. 608ff: Later Victorian Artists.

12 id. Morris, May, p. 618: Decorative Art.

13 id. Traill as above.

14 *Once a Week*, Vol. I, 27 June 1868, p. 119.

15 Meredith, *Diana*, p. 4. (Surrey, ed., 1912.)

16 id. p. 442, '. . . a devious filmy sentimentalist, likely to *fiddle harmonics on the sensual strings* for him at a mad rate for years to come'.

17 id. p. 181.

18 *Nineteenth Century*, January 1883. Reprinted in M. S. Watts, *George Frederick Watts*, p. 203.

19 id. p. 203.

20 id. p. 206.

21 id. p. 207.

22 id. p. 208.

22 id. p. 208.

23 id. p. 210.

24 id. pp. 212 and 213.

25 id. p. 223.

26 id. p. 212.

27 *Daily News*, 1 May 1884.

28 id.

29 id.

30 id. 6 May: 'Dress at the Private Views'.

31 id.

32 id. 7 June.

33 *Patience*, Act I, Lady Jane.

34 *Pall Mall Gazette*, 24 May 1884. From an article called 'Muscle Reading'.

35 *Daily News*, 5 July 1884.
36 Frith, *Autobiography*, Vol. II, p. 256.
37 id.

Chapter 6 SANITARIANS AND WOOLLENERS *pp. 89–114*

 1 *Times*, 8 May 1884. Leader.
 2 *British Medical Journal*, 26 January 1883, p. 187.
 3 *Times*, 12 May 1884.
 4 Godwin, *Dress and its relation to Health and Climate*, p. 1. Pamphlet, 1884.
 5 id. p. 77.
 6 *Lancet*, 10 May 1884, p. 863.
 7 *Times*, 19 May 1884.
 8 *Daily News*, 14 May 1884. Second Leader.
 9 Wilson, *Healthy Life*, p. 194.
10 id. p. 172.
11 *Times*, 26 July 1884. Review of the Health Exhibition's first Hand-
     books.
12 Jaeger, *Health Culture*. Preface, iii.
13 id. Preface, iv.
14 id. p. 44.
15 id. p. 164.
16 id. p. 164.
17 id. p. 168.
18 id. p. 216.
19 *Queen*, August 1878.
20 International Health Exhibition Official Guide.
21 id.
22 King, *Rational Dress*, p. 8.
23 id. p. 16.
24 id. p. 12.
25 id. p. 7.
26 Exhibition of the Rational Dress Association, Catalogue.
27 Ballin, *Science of Dress*, p. 27.
28 id. p. 27.
29 id. p. 178.
30 id. p. 181.
31 id. p. 185.

Chapter 7 NEW ATTITUDES TO REFORM *pp. 115–134*

 1 Rational Dress Society's Gazette. April 1888. 'Item. A Rational
     System of Underclothing'. no page numbers.
 2 id.
 3 id. 'Divided Skirts'.
 4 id. No. 2, October 1888. Editorial Note.
 5 id. p. 4. 'Stays'.

6 *Woman's World*. See, for instance, the editor's 'Note on some Modern Poets' , December 1888, p. 168.
7 id. November 1888, p. 5. 'Shopping in London', by A. E. F. Eliot James.
8 id. May 1888, p. 330. 'May Fashions' by Mrs Johnstone.
9 id. August 1889, p. 482.
10 id. January 1889, p. 283. 'Women wearers of Men's Clothes' by Emily Crawford.
11 id. p. 283ff.
12 id. 1890 Editorial, p. 53ff.
13 id. December 1889, p. 334, 'Notes and Comments'.
14 id. p. 334.
15 id. May 1888, p. 289ff. 'The uses of a Drawing-room' by Henrietta O. Barnet.
16 id. May 1888, p. 374, 'The Society of Lady Dressmakers' by B. A. Cookson-Crackenthorpe.
17 id. June 1888, pp. 337–339. 'Woman and Democracy' by Julia Wedgwood.
18 id. December 1889, p. 390.
19 Ward, *Robert Elsmere*, Vol. I, p. 9.
20 id. Vol. I, p. 314.
21 id. Vol. III, p. 7.
22 id. Vol. II, p. 226.
23 id. Vol. I, p. 10.
24 id. Vol. I, p. 125.
25 *Punch* 1895, drawn by A. S. Boyd. 'A Regular Treat; or, the Radical Tendency'. His Little Lordship – 'Oh, Miss Primsey, I'm going to tell those *nice* boys to come and give us a sail in that *lovely* boat!'
26 Ward, *Robert Elsmere*. Vol. III, p. 257.
27 *Woman's World*, July 1888, p. 415. Children's Dresses in this Century by Mrs Oscar Wilde.
28 id. p. 415.
29 id. p. 417.

Chapter 8 THE ATTACK ON TUBES *pp. 135–148*

1 Jaeger, *Health Culture*, p. 129.
2 id. p. 132.
3 id. p. 136.
4 id. p. 137.
5 id. p. 150.
6 id. p. 153.
7 Harris, *Shaw*, p. 114.
8 Chesterton, *Shaw*, p. 95.
9 *Aglaia*, No. 2, Spring 1894, p. 9.
10 id. p. 13.
11 id. p. 13.

12 id. p. 16.
13 id. p. 19.
14 id. p. 20.
15 id. No. 3, Augumn 1894, p. 13.
16 id. p. 14.
17 id. p. 14.
18 id. p. 35.
19 id. p. 35.
20 Morris, *News from Nowhere*, p. 25.
21 id. pp. 6 and 7.

Chapter 9 Socialist Gowns *pp. 149–167*

1 *Aglaia*, No. 2 on back cover.
2 id.
3 id. No. 1, July 1893, pp. 9 and 10.
4 id. p. 34.
5 id. No. 2, p. 43.
6 id. p. 33.
7 Langley Moore, *Nesbit*, p. 62.
8 id. p. 110. From a description of E. Nesbit by Richard le Gallienne.
9 *Aglaia*, No. 3.
10 id. Advertisement page.
11 Morris, *News from Nowhere*, p. 173.
12 Thompson, *Robert Blatchford; A portrait of an Englishman*, p. 82.
13 *Clarion*, 23 April 1907.
14 *Woman Worker*, No. 1, September 1907.
15 See p. 67 above.
16 *Woman Worker*, September 1907.
17 id. 'The Art of Beauty: The Figure'.
18 id.
19 The sentiments surrounding the early heroes of the Labour Party can be judged from the fact that the lately retired General Secretary of the Trades Union Council, Sir Vic Feather, was named by his parents Victor Grayson Hardie Feather.
20 Harris, *Bernard Shaw*, p. 116–17.

Bibliography

Books and periodicals referred to either directly or indirectly in the text.

BOOKS

ALSTON, A. *The Life and Works of G. F. Watts*. London 1929.

ANON. *Essays in the Defence of Women*. London 1868.

ANON. *Dress, Health and Beauty. A book for ladies containing practical suggestions for the improvement of modern dress regarded from an artistic and sanitary point of view*. London. N.D.

ARNOLD, MATTHEW. *Letters*. 2 vols. ed. George E. Russell, London 1901.

—— *Culture and Anarchy*, London 1869.

—— *Friendship's Garland*, London 1871.

—— *Essays and Letters to Reviews*. Ed. Fraser Neiman. Harvard, Mass. 1960.

—— *Essays in Criticism*. London 1865.

BALLIN, ADA S. *The Science of Dress in theory and practice*. London 1885.

BEALE, L. J., MRCS. *The Laws of Health in relation to Mind and Body*. London 1851.

BLATCHFORD, ROBERT. *Sorcery Shop*. London 1907.

—— *My Eighty Years*. London 1931.

BLOOMER, D. C. *The Life and Writings of Amelia Bloomer*. Boston, Mass. 1895.

BRADDON, M. E. *Lady Audley's Secret*. London 1862.

—— *Asphodel*. London.

BRUCE, MARY. *Anna Swanwick*. London 1903.

BURNET, FRANCES HODGSON. *Little Lord Fauntleroy*. London 1888.

BURTON, HESTER. *Barbara Bodichon*. London 1949.

BUSS, GEORG. *Das Kostum*. Leipzig 1906.

CAPLIN, ROXEY A. *Health and Beauty in Woman and her Clothing*. London 1864.

CHESTERTON, G. K. *George Bernard Shaw*. London 1910.

CHRISTIE, C. F. *The Transition from Aristocracy 1832–67*. London 1927.

COMBE, ANDREW, M.D. *The principles of physiology applied to the preservation of Health and to the improvement of physical and mental Education. 1834*. 14th edition. ed. James Coxe, MD. London 1852.

COOK, SIR EDWARD. *Florence Nightingale*. 2 vols. London 1913.

CRANE, LUCY. *Art and the formation of Taste*. London 1882.

CRANE, WALTER. *The First of May: a fairy masque presented in a series of 52 designs by Walter Crane*. London 1881.

—— *Pan-pipes. A Book of Old Songs*. London nd.

—— *The claims of Decorative Art*. London 1892.

—— *Preface to Embroidery or the Craft of the Needle*. London & New York 1899.

—— *May Day 1903*. Socialist Festival Souvenir. Cover by Walter Crane.

Bibliography

DISRAELI, B. *Lothair.* ed. London 1881.

DOUGLAS, MRS. *The Gentlewoman's Book of Dress.* London nd.

FRITH, W. P. *My Autobiography and Reminiscences.* London 1887.

GILBERT, W. S. *The Savoy Operas,* Vol. I. ed. London 1962.

GRAVES, CHARLES L. *Mr Punch's History of Modern England,* 4 vols. London 1921.

HALÉVY, ELIE. *History of the English People, Epilogue 1895–1905,* 2 vols. ed. London 1939.

HARRIS, FRANK. *Bernard Shaw.* London 1931.

HAWEIS, MRS. *The Art of Dress.* London 1878.

—— *The Art of Decoration.* London 1881.

HOWE, BEA. *Arbiter of Elegance.* London 1967.

HUNT, W. HOLMAN. *PreRaphaelitism and the PreRaphaelite Brotherhood,* 2 vols. London 1905.

JAEGER, GUSTAVE. *Essays in Health Culture.* London 1887.

KING, E. M. *Rational Dress or, the Dress of Women and Savages.* London 1882.

'LIMNER, LUKE ESQ.' *Madre Nature versus the Moloch of Fashion.* London 1874.

LINTON, MRS LYNN. *The Girl of the Period.* London 1884.

MACKMURDO, A. H. ED. *Plain Handicrafts.* Preface by G. F. Watts: articles by Lethaby, May Morris, Selwyn Image. London 1892.

MCGRIGOR, ALLAN J. *Woman Suffrage Wrong.* London 1892.

MEREDITH, GEORGE. *Diana of the Crossways.* London 1885. Surrey ed. 1912.

MERRIFIELD, MRS. *Dress as a Fine Art.* London 1854.

MILL, JOHN STUART. *The Subjection of Women.* London 1869.

MILLAIS, JOHN GUILLE. *The Life and Letters of Sir John Everett Millais,* 2 vols. London 1899.

MOORE, DORIS LANGLEY. *E. Nesbit.* London 1933.

MORRIS, WILLIAM. *News from Nowhere.* London 1891.

NICHOLS, T. L. *Human Psychology.* London 1872.

NIELSON, CHARLES. *The Bloomer Girls.* London 1967.

OLIPHANT, MRS. *At his Gates,* 3 vols. London 1872.

—— *Carita,* 3 vols. London 1877.

PUDOR, H. *Frauer Reform Kleidung.* Leipzig 1903.

'R'. *Dress in a Nutshell.* London 1901.

READE, CHARLES. *Christie Johnstone.* London 1853.

—— *The Course of True Love Never Did Run Smooth.* London 1897.

ROSSETTI, DANTE GABRIEL. *Letters.* ed. O. Doughty and J. R. Wake, vol. I. Oxford 1965.

RUSKIN, JOHN. *The Crown of Wild Olive.* London 1866.

SHAW, G. B. *Caesar and Cleopatra.* London 1901.

STANTON, THEODORE, ED. *The Woman Question in Europe,* a series of essays. London 1884.

STEPHEN, BARBARA. *Emily Davies and Girton College.* London 1927.

STRACHEY, ROY. *Millicent Fawcett.* London 1931.

SURTEES, VIRGINIA. *The Paintings and Drawings of Dante Gabriel Rossetti,* 2 vols. Oxford 1971.

TEIRLINCK, HERMAN. *Henry van der Velde.* Brussels 1959.
THOMPSON, LAURENCE. *Robert Blatchford; a portrait of an Englishman.* London 1951.
TOWNSEND, W. G. PAULSON. *Embroidery or the Craft of the Needle.* Preface by Walter Crane. London and New York 1899.
TRAILL, H. D. and MANN, J. S. ed. *Social England 1801–1895,* vol. 6. London 1901–4.
WARD, MRS HUMPHREY. *Robert Elsmere,* 3 vols. London 1888. ed. 1901 1, vol.
WATTS, M. S. *George Frederick Watts,* 3 vols. London 1912.
WILSON, GEORGE, MD. *Healthy Life and Healthy Dwellings.* London 1880.
YONGE, CHARLOTTE. *Three Brides.* London 1876. ed. 1904.

NEWSPAPERS AND PERIODICALS

Aglaia. London, 1893–94
Atalanta. London, October 1893–September 1894.
British Medical Journal. 1883–84.
Clarion, The. London, 1907–08.
Costume, the Journal of the Costume Society, Vol. VII, 1973. 'Bonnard's Costume Historique – a Pre-Raphaelite Source Book' by Roger Smith.
Daily News, The. London, January–August 1884.
Edinburgh Review, The. Edinburgh, 1862.
Fortnightly Review, The London. August–November 1865. January–June 1884.
Graphic, The. London, 1874 and 1884.
Illustrated London News, The. London 1884.
Kettledrum, The. London, 1869.
Lancet, The. London, 1874 and 1883–84.
Leisure. Dublin, 1869.
Macmillan's Magazine. London, 1869.
Nineteenth Century, The. London, 1880, 1883, 1884.
Once-a-Week. London, January 1868–August 1870.
Owl, The. London, January–June 1864. January–June 1868.
Owlet Papers, The. London, 1861.
Pall Mall Gazette, The. London, 1868–69.
Punch. London, 1853–59. 1868. 1875. 1884. 1888. 1890–99.
Queen, The. London, 1875–78.
Rational Dress Society's Gazette. London, 1888–89.
Saturday Review, The. London, 1868.
Times, The. London, March–June 1868. October–December 1883. January–August 1884.
Woman. London, 1890.
Woman Worker, The. London, 1907–10.
Woman's World, The. London, I, 1868, II, 1888–90.

CATALOGUES

Exhibition of the Rational Dress Association, Princes Hall 1883.

Bibliography

International Health Exhibition, Kensington. Official Guide 1884.
Shakespearean Show, Kensington 1884.
Royal Academy, Bicentary Exhibition, Burlington House 1969.

MISCELLANEOUS
The Builder, Pamphlets on Art, 1884.
Hansard.
Poetical Broadsides, Collection British Museum nd.
Evolution in Costume, compiled and invented by Messrs Liberty, revised ed.
  January 1894.

Index

Names of persons in inverted commas indicate
that they are characters in novels.

Index